Occupational Therapy in Short-term Psychiatry

Moya Willson BA TDip COT
Senior Lecturer, Salford School of Occupational Therapy

CHURCHILL LIVINGSTONE
EDINBURGH LONDON MELBOURNE AND NEW YORK 1984

CHURCHILL LIVINGSTONE
Medical Division of Longman Group UK Limited

Distributed in the United States of America by Churchill
Livingstone Inc., 1560 Broadway, New York, N.Y.
10036, and by associated companies, branches and
representatives throughout the world.

First published 1984
  Reprinted 1985
  Reprinted 1987

ISBN 0-443-02921-0

British Library Cataloguing in Publication Data
Willson, Moya
  Occupational therapy in short-term psychiatry.
  1. Occupational therapy
  I. Title
  616.89'1652   RC487

Library of Congress Cataloging in Publication Data
Main entry under title:
Occupational therapy in short-term psychiatry.
  Includes index.
  1. Occupational therapy — Addresses, essays,
lectures. 2. Psychotherapy, Brief — Addresses, essays,
lectures. I. Willson, Moya. [DNLM: 1. Occupational
therapy. 2. Mental disorders — Therapy. 3. Psychotherapy,
Brief. WM 450.5.02]
RC487.027 1984 616.89'165 84-3156

Produced by Longman Group (FE) Ltd
Printed in Hong Kong

Preface

This book is intended to assist occupational therapists and their students who are working in, or learning about, general psychiatry. The client group referred to includes those with a wide range of disorders which should not normally give rise to long-term care. Little emphasis has been given to classification on the basis of clinical signs and symptoms. A broader approach to unhappiness and disadvantage should be relevant to therapists who are primarily concerned with helping people to resolve individual difficulties in living. This presupposes, in each reader, a basic knowledge of psychology, sociology and psychiatry, or at least that these subjects are being studied concurrently.

The first section of the book discusses the variety of problems which may lead to referral. The chapters on mental illness and the vulnerable personality require no explanation. The inclusion of a chapter on physical disability may surprise those who have forgotten that to draw artificial lines between mental and physical health is, potentially, to deny clients on either side a full and flexible programme of treatment.

The second section selects three topics which I feel to be of particular significance to this area of practice. The first is humanistic psychology, popular with many therapists as a baseline for thinking and for action. The other two topics, attitudes and social competence, are linked with each other and are the two concepts which therapists, knowingly or unknowingly, apply to almost every problem. These three chapters are intended to identify some particular influences on the way in which therapy is devised and presented, appreciating that there are many other factors which should also be taken into account.

The third section is more practically oriented and describes what occupational therapists may actually do. The chapters on social skills training, the management of anxiety, and creative therapies are based on specific techniques. Those on constructive activities, leisure and strategic skills offer the background of concern and activity essential to an integrated service.

No book on occupational therapy, or any other form of therapy in psychiatry, can claim to be comprehensive. Too much is unknown and the problems of individuals must be regarded as being unique. As in any other field of knowledge it is important to recognise both what you know and also what you do not know. One of the exciting things about working in psychiatry is that many different ideas, interpretations and techniques can be applied to the practical problems with which one is presented. There is space and opportunity for sensitivity, problem solving and innovation. There is also a responsibility involved in being allowed, by society, to intervene in the lives of other people. This should not be taken lightly. A diploma to practise and a few good ideas gleaned from this or any other book do not entitle one to take risks with the well-being of others. Any experimental projects should be carefully conceived and well documented; any help that you can offer is not a privilege to the recipient.

The contributors to this book have each offered different ideas, knowledge and skills. I would like to thank each of them for their time, willingness and enthusiasm, and hope that credit is given to those who have done the work. The final manuscript was only produced through the expert secretarial assistance of Celeste Wright who types and retypes with unfailing good humour, and who should not be one of the unsung heroines of our times.

Salford, 1984   Moya Willson

Contributors

Lesley Carter DipCOT

Elizabeth Cracknell BSc TDipCOT
Director of Training, School of Occupational Therapy, St Andrew's Hospital, Northampton

Barbara Cullen DipCOT
Occupational Therapist, Metropolitan Borough of Knowsley Social Services

Diana Grellier TDipCOT
Head of Salford School of Occupational Therapy, Salford

Christine M. Hewitt TDipCOT
Senior Lecturer, Ulster Polytechnic, Jordanstown

Joan King TDipCOT
Vice Principal, Dorset House School of Occupational Therapy, Oxford

Margaret Nicol TDipCOT
Lecturer in Occupational Therapy, Queen Margaret College, Edinburgh

Christine Ravetz BA DipCOT
Lecturer in Occupational Therapy, Salford College of Technology, Salford

Averil M. Steward FCOT TDip
Senior Lecturer in Occupational Therapy, Queen Margaret College, Edinburgh

Rose Stockwell BSc(Hons) DipCOT
Senior Occupational Therapist, Atkinson Morley's Hospital, Wimbledon

Michael Willson BSc MA
Consultant in Social Work Management

Contributors

Contents

The clients

The clients

Mental illness

INTRODUCTION

Mental illness is a precarious topic. Even a cursory glance at past and present literature reveals it to be the subject of passionate debate. Some of the views held are so opposed that they seem never to penetrate further than problems of definition, and the battlefield becomes one of semantics.

This chapter does not seek to uphold or condemn any particular frame of reference but rather describes the subject and its debate. The emphasis is on the description and disabilities of those who are perceived by others to be 'sick' or 'mad'. An alternative social view of the inability of some people to cope within society is the subject of the next chapter, although it is inevitable that a high degree of overlap occurs.

The word madman is no longer used to describe someone who has a disordered mind. Likewise lunatic, maniac, bedlamite, raver and idiot are terms which have changed their meaning as knowledge and attitudes have claimed greater sophistication. Interestingly, these have all become terms which have a dual purpose of abuse and endearment, depending on the context in which they are used.

If normality or sanity could be defined and understood as a baseline against which abnormality could be measured, then the study of psychiatry would be much easier. As it is, many people now avoid the use of 'normal' or 'sane' in description for fear of being challenged to explain what they mean. Depression, anxiety, anti-social behaviour, addiction, delusion and confusion are all normal features in that they may be represented within the life span of a person who functions adequately, or at least does not appeal for help. These are all also symptoms of abnormality when they are present to an incapacitating degree, or when they are recognised in a person who is failing to cope with his life. It may be useful to use the term 'average' rather than 'normal' to describe those who do not come to the attention of professional agencies. Their experience of the world does not cross that line beyond which one does not only worry about oneself but is *worried about* by other people, who ultimately act.

Being outside the average range gives rise to being exceptional. Consider this statement in relation to physical health:

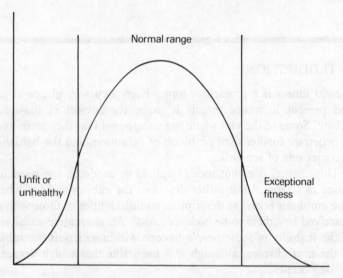

Fig. 1.1 A simplified distribution curve related to physical fitness.

A second very simplified curve shows the same concept applied to mental health. Note that, for convenience, neither diagram includes the bulge of infirmity which is the result of physical accidents.

This seems terribly obvious until one starts wondering why the two vertical lines, which form the boundaries of normal range, are placed where they are. In the diagrams they were placed arbitrarily in order to illustrate a point; in reality they move according to cultural, economic and political pressures. The reasons why these boundary lines move, making the normal range more or less inclusive, include the following.

1. *The resources of the community which can be directed towards health or social services.* In parts of the world where survival and physical health are threatened there is less emphasis on recognising and aiding those who are psychologically disturbed. There also may be less effort made to identify and exploit the strengths of those

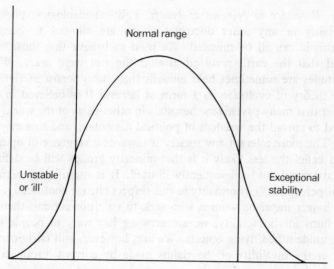

Normal range

Unstable
or 'ill'

Exceptional
stability

Fig. 1.2 The same concept applied to mental stability.

who are exceptional at the positive end of the scale. On the other hand, wealthy nations or communities can direct more resources to fulfilling the needs of their exceptional members and hence can afford to diagnose more people as being ill in some way. Note that the 'incidence' of any disorder is calculated on the number of times it is diagnosed and may not be a true reflection of the number of people who may be experiencing its effects.

2. *The acceptability of diagnosis and treatment.* Both doctors and their patients are subject to social controls when they seek to define the situation which they are in. On an international level, for example, the diagnosis of schizophrenia is more inclusive in some parts of the world than in others (World Health Organization, 1972). Individually, many psychiatrists are becoming more sensitive to the negative effects of diagnostic labelling and are more reluctant to define a patient as not belonging within a normal range of human behaviour and distress. On a social level the negative effects of stigma may lead to different patterns of self-referral for help. National attitudes and social class are both influential. To give two extremes, in some subcultures a regular appointment with a psychoanalyst or membership of a therapeutic group is almost a mark of sensitive respectability. In another, a disabling degree of emotional distress may only give rise to a belated visit to a general practitioner on the pretext of some related physical complaint.

3. *Reference to opinions or beliefs.* Political ideologies, popular morality or any other doctrines which are allowed to become dogmatic can all be misused. We used to believe that those who held that the earth revolved around the sun were crazy. What attitudes are sometimes held towards those who persist in viewing the theory of evolution as a form of heresy? It is believed in the West that many psychiatric hospitals in other parts of the world are used to curtail the freedom of political dissenters, and this may be so. The more tolerant any society is towards divergence of opinion and belief the less likely it is that minority groups will be defined as abnormal, and subsequently ill-used. It is useful to remember that perceptions of normality in this respect change continually. We no longer imprison women who seek to vote nor commit them to asylums for immorality; we are growing less wary of people who see unidentified flying objects. We are, however, still fairly certain about the invalidity of the claims made by current 'prophets' or 'messiahs'.

4. *The variability of social support.* This is a difficult one and may be a confusing addition, but it does have great significance to those who exist very close to that wobbling vertical line. Individuals who are referred for treatment, by either themselves or others, are often those who are without close friends or relatives or whose family dynamics are a part of the problem. The tendency towards a social structure of nuclear rather than extended families may throw the weak or the peculiar into sharper relief. The frustrations of poverty or unemployment may cement family relationships, may create emotional disorder or may lay bare a previously supported member of the family who can no longer be tolerated. Variations in social support are closely influenced by the previous three points. However, many individuals who share the same apparent degree of incapacity or stress can be identified on different sides of the defining line. The difference between them is the amount of social support which they receive from family or friends.

PSYCHIATRY AND REALITY

Problems of description

Psychiatric disorders are categories which have been invented by psychiatrists. Such categories are usually inclusive of a number of problems and personal circumstances which are frequently found in conjunction with each other. For example, symptoms which include misery, sleep disturbance, pre-occupation with bowel function and general retardation, found in conjunction with the menopause and with changes in responsibility, could be recognised by some as being a syndrome. A syndrome is something one has seen before and will probably see again.

It is not, however, always possible to place a whole range of physical, emotional or cognitive experiences along one axis of an imaginary grid, place typical features of personality and biography along the other and identify specific disorders in the way that the mileage between destinations can be found on the chart at the back of a road atlas.

If each psychiatric disorder had a number of unmistakable features, which did not grossly overlap with those belonging to other disorders, then it would be possible to use the study of plants as a parallel. By general examination the family could be established and by closer scrutiny the individual species identified. Some organically based problems, for example both amentia and dementia, will admit such a parallel to a large degree. Other areas of psychiatric concern are either less advanced or more complex than the study of botany. In some cases we can identify the family but are less sure about the species. This might apply to 'schizophrenia'. In other conditions, for example anorexia nervosa, the description of the disorder is precise enough to think that it is a species but there is room for disagreement about the family to which it belongs.

Diseases of the mind

The word disease ought to cause few problems since it has been applied precisely within physical medicine for a very long time. Within psychiatry, however, it provides a useful example of apparent disagreements or confusions which may bother (or stimulate) a student who is new to the subject. Compare the following statements:

Silvano Arieti (1978): 'If "disease" means a condition that causes a dysfunction of the organism, irrespective of evidence of cellular pathology and irrespective of the nature of the cause which determined it, we can certainly call depression a disease.'

Christian Scharfetter (1980): 'In psychiatry the medical model of *illness* can be used only in those mental disorders which are associated with physical illness (especially cerebral disease): acute exogenous reactions, amnestic psychodramas, the dementias, the organic psychoses (brain syndromes).'

Jeff Coulter (1973): 'Why should we think that those phenomena to which we intelligibly refer with the word 'disease' should manifest invariant, common properties that we could codify neatly into a list or a definition . . . . . It seems to me that much of the ink that is wasted in constructing definitions of 'disease' derives from the attempt in psychopathology to rationalize the use of the medical nosology'.

Incidentally, the word nosology means the study of classification of disorders and the word 'psychiatry', according to the Concise Oxford Dictionary means 'study and treatment of mental disease'. Now read these two personal accounts written by two young people admitted to an acute psychiatric admission unit.

Young woman of 28:

There isn't anything inside me, there isn't anything to feel. I'm not sad because I am not anything and you should not come to me because of the stench . . . . . because only my bowels are full and I feel that I am rotting. I don't want to eat any more, food will only sustain the badness. You cannot reach me because I have to be alone and I cannot get out because I'm sorry for all the things I've done. Sorry for them, not sorry for me—and you should not be because there is nothing. I have slipped away from myself but my body drags on and anchors my sin.

17-year-old youth:

It all started to happen last year one summer and I have had it to this day. That is why I am writing a diary of the action.

1. It first started last summer with worry and strange thoughts. It came to me gradually. It just affected me by making me think that people were putting their worries and problems on to me and leaving their badness on me and on the furniture such as chairs, doors, knives, forks and spoons, money etc. and if I touched them I would get all their worries and problems.
2. Then I thought that people were taking my sight in some way such as if I looked at a book and and turned the page over I thought I had left some of my sight there on the page I was looking at.
3. And if somebody bumped into me or touched me I felt that they were taking my goodness.
4. Or if I was walking along a road and a bus or a car or a person walked past I felt that they were taking part of my body with them. The same thing happened if I walked or ran past a lamp post and I could really feel this strange force taking place.
5. Some time after this sickness I had other thoughts. I felt I was walking on people or on my pet fish. Then one day one of my

best fish died. Could this have something to do with what I was thinking? Other things like this happened.

6. Then another thought came. People and places played on my mind and when I thought of a place I felt as if I was going there in spirit and seeing it as it was at that time. Then I thought people were voodooing me and caused things to happen to me and my home.

7. Then I thought everyone was against me. I thought people would rob my thoughts, my sight, my strength and I thought I had a number and if anybody knew that number which is number 12 they would break me, and I thought if I thought of anything at home or anything at all people could see and hear what I was thinking and if I didn't jump up and bless myself they could hear and see what I am thinking. I felt people could rob my ears and if I throw any rubbish away I was throwing my goodness with it and when I walked I felt I was draining out. I stopped this from happening by jumping up and down and blessing myself or going back and touching things, or closing my eyes and getting my sight back from other people. I went to have my eyes tested. They were alright but I still had these things happening to me.

I stopped going out and stopped reading and watching telly. One day when I got round to reading I saw a column about O.B.E. out of body experience where people can leave their bodies in spirit.

What a coincidence I thought could this be true, could this be happening to me?

So I am still troubled with these thoughts but I have learned to live with them and I am better now. All the same these things are still on my mind—they could be true.

Having registered their distress we can continue to 'waste ink' in discussing the general concept of disease or we can state that there is something *wrong* with them in comparison with other people and not worry too much about semantics. Neither course of action would be satisfactory since one needs to be able to describe a problem with some confidence before attempting to deal with it.

The way in which different doctors or therapists describe problems is dependent on their previous experience, their education and their beliefs. The next section will therefore summarise several of the different viewpoints which may influence their perceptions of abnormality.

Differing perspectives

In the past, explanations of deviancy were derived from beliefs then held and knowledge then available. Hence the acceptance that it was possible to be possessed by demons or that individuals could be guilty of witchcraft. As an alternative to demonology early somatogenic theories proposed physical factors which supposedly directed both personality and also aberrant behaviour. These are mentioned in Chapter 2.

Within current thinking demonology has given way to the more scientifically based studies of psychology and human relationships. Somatology has matured into a highly sophisticated understanding of how human physiology may influence human behaviour.

The current perspectives, derived from this historical background, are the psychodynamic, the behavioural and learning, the humanistic and the physiological.

The psychodynamic

Also known as the psychoanalytical approach, the concepts derive from theories of personality. Historically the most influential figure in this field is Sigmund Freud. Students of occupational therapy should be aware of the way in which he described mental structures including the roles of the *id, ego* and *superego* in directing the personality on both conscious and unconscious levels. Personality theorists place a great deal of emphasis on development and the significance of early trauma or deprivation. Freud describes oral, anal, phallic, latent and genital phases, each of which presents conflicts. The manner in which these conflicts are resolved, or fail to be resolved, influences future pathology in the adult. In Freudian terms, psychological problems are described as fixations and complexes. A fixation, for example anal fixation, denotes a blockage in development which leaves the individual frozen or 'fixed' at a stage in psychosexual development and still seeking the appropriate gratification. Complexes arise from the genital phase and relate to sexual attraction to either parent figure. Hence the terms 'Oedipus complex' in the male and 'Electra complex' in the female. Freud also described neurotic anxiety which may be 'free-floating' as experienced within phobias or as 'panic reactions' which are more transient in experience but equally deep rooted. A failure to resolve developmental conflicts or to deal with anxiety on a conscious level gives rise to defence mechanisms. These include repression, projection, displacement, reaction formation, regression and rationalisation, several of which are described within Chapter 2.

The ideas of Freud, and those who developed and expanded his work and who are known as 'neo-Freudians', form the basis of individual and group psychotherapy today. Those who adhere to their concepts will seek the explanation for present distress in the biography of the patient and his ability to reveal unconscious material through techniques such as 'free association'. They will translate therapeutic relationships in terms of positive and negative transference and be sensitive to the likelihood of 'projection' when the patient describes relationships, objects or events. Some of these terms may be unfamiliar but they will not be defined or discussed further here since they are well documented. Essentially, it should be understood that personality theorists offer an interpretation, which relates to the past, to current experiences of distress or stagnation. Projective techniques, such as the Thematic Apperception and the Rorschach Ink Blot tests are the tools of analysts who work within this frame of reference and are not normally utilised by occupational therapists. Creative activities, using various art forms discussed within Chapter 9, may serve as an adjunct to a psychodynamic approach to treatment. They may assist a patient to identify, and come to terms with, events or emotions which are significant within his own biography and relationships.

Behavioural and learning

Theorists of this persuasion tell us that all behaviour is learnt and hence problems can be described in terms of inappropriate learning or of failure to learn. When problems or anxieties arise, most people adopt strategies which are reasonably successful and which do not, in themselves, give rise to further problems. A tendency to adopt the wrong strategies, or to be socially helpless or inadequate, can be recognised in many individuals who are described as having psychological disorders. More extreme pieces of behaviour, such as social withdrawal, autism and bizarre or confused speech can be seen as an attempt to escape from personal and social difficulties.

Behaviourists base their descriptions of behaviour, and their attempts to modify it, on the experimental findings of psychologists who have studied learning. Early influences were, of course, Ivan Pavlov who described classical conditioning, and Edward Thorndyke, followed by Frederick Skinner who laid down the foundations of operant conditioning. An appreciation of the types of learning involved in classical conditioning enabled clinicians to develop methods such as desensitisation and aversion in order to change the response made by an individual to a given set of stimuli. Strategies arising from operant conditioning, such as token economy and bio-feedback, are used to elicit behaviour from a subject in order to gain a desired response.

More recently learning theorists have become interested in the social context in which learning takes place. Modelling, as a teaching technique, has emerged from experimental work which demonstrates that watching someone else perform a task, or fulfil a social role, enables the observer to acquire complex patterns of behaviour before active involvement has taken place. Children, of course, learn much of their repetoire of social behaviour in this way (see Ch. 7). It should be remembered that it is not just observable behaviour which is subject to imitative learning. Attitudes and anxieties can be conveyed from one 'generation' to another by the omission or discouragement of discussion and activity. There is, for example, little opportunity within western society to witness adult sexual behaviour. However, the conditioned emotional responses of parents to sexual stimuli appear to be transmitted to their children. A study of aggressive and inhibited boys (Bandura, 1960) indicated that parents who were anxious about sex tended to have sons who experienced guilt in relation to sex and who had difficulty in establishing close, affectionate friendships. Davison and Neale (1982) suggest that 'of all the aspects of human suffering that command the attention of psychopathologists and clinicians, few touch the lives of more people than problems involving sex'. Many psychosexual disorders are perceived to stem from early learning and socialisation, treatment being offered ranging from aversion to social skills training.

An interest in social learning also leads to the study of personal and social perception. The cognitive structure within which a person thinks about himself, other people and events will determine the style and effectiveness of his behaviour. A structure which leads to feelings of helplessness or inadequacy may be a part of the picture presented by someone who is depressed (see Ch. 2). Therapists who have tried to apply these ideas within treatment refer to the need for *cognitive restructuring*. This involves suggesting to a patient alternative and positive ways of describing to himself what is happening or what events mean. For example, statements such as 'it does not matter if I fail as long as I know that I did my best', or 'I believe I am able to control the children's behaviour', can be rehearsed and invoked to help an individual to act in a more positive way when feeling stressed.

The perspectives applied by a behaviourally oriented clinician to the problems of a client may be based on some or all of these ideas. Essentially he will be interested in the behaviour, its immediate antecedents and its consequences. This interest may extend to identifying current beliefs and attitudes which determine how someone will experience and respond to events.

The humanistic or existential view

Those who follow the lead given by Maslow and Rogers place stress on reality as it is experienced by the client. In order to share this reality a clinician must learn to empathise, or to adopt the other's phenomenological frame of reference. These terms are explained within Chapter 4 which is devoted to this topic because of its particular significance to occupational therapy.

Gestalt therapy, as described by Fritz Perls (1951), extends these ideas but differs slightly in its special emphasis on the present. Immediate experience and the comfortable satisfaction of current needs are made important; changes in behaviour are made by enhancing what an individual does and says and helping him to accept responsibility for these expressions.

Clinicians who are influenced by these ideas will be alert to the client's presentation of self, will be sensitive to freedom of will and expression, and will encourage self-determination. Solutions to problems are sought from within the client and not sought elsewhere in order to be prescribed.

The physiological view

Here we come full circle to the concept of disease which was used earlier as an example of difficulties in descriptive terms. Terminology is important since the use, within psychiatry, of words associated with physical medicine influences the way in which we think about people and their problems. Maher (1966) demonstrates this very neatly by stating that: '(deviant) behaviour is termed *pathological* and is classified on the basis of *symptoms*, classification being called *diagnosis*. Processes designed to change behaviour are called *therapies* and are applied to patients in mental *hospitals*. If the deviant behaviour ceases, the patient is described as *cured*.'

Attempting to categorise people on the basis of their behaviour, their descriptions of how they think and feel and their personal history is difficult. The presence of any physical abnormality introduces a welcome degree of objectivity into the assessment which is being made. A physiological or medical approach describes distress as being the result of illness which, once identified, should be amenable to treatment. Strict adherance to this model assumes that conditions in which physiological abnormalities have not yet been discovered have been incompletely researched. Once the congenital abnormality, the virus, the traumatic damage or the chemical deficiency has been identified then the appropriate treatment can be developed.

It is very easy to criticise this 'medical' model of abnormal behaviour, indeed it is almost fashionable to do so. Here are examples of the types of ammunition which might be used:

'When a disease model is applied to abnormal behaviour (however) it is often not possible to assess independently both the symptoms and the supposed cause of the symptoms. Certain behaviour or symptoms are categorised as mental illnesses and given names, but then the name of the illness itself is often cited as an explanation for or cause of these same symptoms. For example, a patient who is withdrawn and hallucinating is diagnosed as schizophrenic; however, when we ask why the patient is withdrawn and hallucinating, we are often told that it is because the patient is schizophrenic' (Davison and Neale, 1982).

Or, in somewhat terser tone look at this suggestion made by Coulter (1973):

'Biogenic theorists of the aetiology of mental disorder cannot hope to achieve a statement of the necessary and sufficient conditions for the holding of some bizarre belief or the communication of some unusual experiences.'

On the other hand, physiological psychiatry has an undeniable track record. The treatment of endocrine and metabolic disorders which used to lead to mental handicap are now recognised and treated. General Paralysis of the Insane has become a historic interest rather than a current problem. Genetic counselling is available to those who risk endangering their offspring with genetically transmitted forms of presenile dementia.

Examples of a second level of success can be seen in the control, by physical means, of psychological distress. Minor group tranquillisers, antidepressant and hallucinogenic drugs allow people to start to tackle problems again. Phenothiazine derivatives appear to make endurable the more bizarre aspects of psychosis or otherwise uncontrolled anxiety. Electroconvulsive treatment, more controversially, relieves states of depression in some people. These successes are rated as secondary for two main reasons. The first is that they ameliorate but do not cure and in some cases the reasons for their effectiveness are not fully understood. Secondly they do not admit a possible 'chicken and egg' problem within psychiatry; do physiological abnormalities in the transmission of nerve impulses, which may be a feature of depressive illness, precede the disturbance of mood or are they a consequence of it? Are the abnormal levels of cortical arousal part of a pattern of malfunction which causes 'schizophrenic' behaviour or do they arise from some other more significant distress? The answers proposed to such questions are not quite convincing enough yet.

Another criticism of the medical model is that it is more use to doctors and research workers than to patients and to other disciplines which seek to offer help. It gives rise to problems of diagnostic labelling without prescribing a clear course of ameliorative action. The worst tags are those such as 'personality disorder' which define abnormality in vague and abstract terms. The problem is retained in the province of medicine but physiological abnormalities are not sought with any vigour in the jungle of biographical disasters and personal failures.

Recapitulation

This chapter has so far failed to define mental illness but has posed some questions. It is hoped that these questions are more pertinent to a student of occupational therapy than a list of facts for easy memorisation would have been. This may sound like an excuse, but the most important thing that a professional education can give to you is an opportunity to join in the debate, to compare different viewpoints and to develop your own working philosophy. In order to do this an occupational therapist must have a working knowledge of clinical psychiatry; a useful summary is not given here since many excellent textbooks are available. It is also essential to be able to apply knowledge about psychology to a function–dysfunction continuum and to integrate ideas from other disciplines, in particular sociology, into an understanding of what may be going on.

PRACTICAL PROBLEMS

Occupational therapists seek to assist people in practical ways. They are interested in the skills which an individual is able to draw upon when performing everyday tasks and also in the concepts and attitudes which affect his performance of roles. Occupational therapy is essentially a social process which is problem oriented. Its practitioners do not normally prescribe forms of activity or therapy on the basis of symptom or diagnosis.

There are a number of subjective experiences which are shared by a wide variety of clients and which contribute to their difficulties in both task and role performance. They tend, also, to be the experiences which are active in preventing the client from sharing perceptions of the social world with others, thereby excluding him from the personal contacts which arise out of a shared reality. Three important areas in which these experiences occur are disorders of perception, disorders of thought and disturbance of mood. It is difficult to think of any psychological disorder which does not involve at least one of these.

Disorders of perception

The process of perception involves organising and interpreting sensory stimuli. It is relatively straightforward if you think of it purely as a part of receiving information about the environment. Visual perception, for example, involves the translation of the retinal image of the object in my hand to the 'knowledge' that it is a black pen. Sensory inputs from other receptors are also translated and add to my current perception that the pen is light, warm and makes a noise as it travels across the paper. Using this level of description we can accept the definition of a hallucination as being a perception in the absence of any relevant external stimuli. Thus a visual hallucination involves 'seeing' something which is not physically present and an auditory hallucination hearing something although no sound is discernible by others. Hallucinations may involve any of the sensory modalities. Some people report 'combined' hallucinations where more than one sense is involved but it would be unusual to report not only seeing a pink elephant but also smelling, tasting, touching and hearing it.

It is important to differentiate between hallucinations and illusions. The latter are a misinterpretation or 'misperception' of sensory information which is actually present. An everyday example would be a mirage, perceiving a pool of water on the road ahead when actually the visual information should have been interpreted as a combination of heat haze and the reflection of sun on tarmac. It is not the eye that is fooled but the brain, and psychologists spend hours producing pictures and models to demonstrate the extent to which we can be misled in our perceptions of perspective, distance, depth, colour and size.

The problem of describing perception, and then hallucination and illusion, as an extension of the sensory modalities is that this oversimplifies the process in a way which can be misleading in itself. Perception is an active process which includes the involvement of memory, expectations and mood, and attention as well as other factors not expanded upon here.

Recall

It is quite obvious that in order to identify a stimulus we compare it with information that has been 'stored' about previous experiences. This is not necessarily a conscious process. I can recognise my back door key amongst others on a ring but could not 'bring to mind' and describe its position on the ring, the shape of its indentations or the number engraved on it. I know it is a key, that is I can place it in a generalised family of different shaped objects all called keys, and I know that it is my back door key because I can select its own particular features. What is more I can do it in the dark. All cognition must necessarily involve re-cognition. It is likely that the process is one of testing any novel pattern of stimuli against a series of hypotheses, actively searching for a reasonable interpretation.

Expectation and mood

We frequently see or hear that which we were expecting. This is one of the major reasons why we can be taken in by illusions. Geometrical illusions to be found in psychology textbooks often mislead us by using previous experiences of perspective or relative sizes and shapes in a context where they do not apply.

There is, however, another way in which expectations can affect perception. We can associate certain environments or situations with the likelihood of pleasant or unpleasant experiences. Walking down a dark street at night, with the knowledge of frightening things that have happened to others in just such a setting, how are you likely to perceive a sudden movement in the shadows or a light clicking noise? Escalating anxiety, and then panic, in such a situation can lead to seeing, hearing or feeling things which do not exist.

One's prevalent mood can also distort perception, or at least lead one's perceptions of the world to be out of tune with the perceptions of others. Scharfetter (1980) suggests that 'In depression, to a severely downcast and melancholy man his surroundings seem less lively, colourful, clear and distinct. Sometimes, it is as though he were experiencing them at a distance. A depressed patient may experience himself as falling to pieces; feeling putrefied, he may even smell the decayed odour that eminates from him'.

Attention

Accurate perception and the organisation of sensory input is reliant on some degree of selective attention to stimuli. To perceive every stimulus available to you simultaneously would be overwhelming and would result in not being able to give meaning to the environment at all. However, in order to select out certain stimuli which are to be perceived, it must be necessary to recognise all of them and to discard the irrelevant. This is illustrated by the well known 'cocktail party phenomenon', when you selectively attend to one conversation and are unaware of the content of others until your own name is mentioned. Whatever mechanism has been censoring out irrelevant stimuli has recognised a significant input and sent it up for attention. There has been considerable research in this field since Broadbent (1958) suggested the existence of an active filtering mechanism. Students of occupational therapy should pay particular attention to factors which may be responsible for the apparently anarchic experience of the world as perceived by those with 'psychotic conditions'. If a wide range of stimuli are competing for attention, and if we accept that some are selected and others determined to be irrelevant, then this raises important questions about the criteria used by any individual for the selection of relevant material. Both the interests and the mood of an individual will influence his selective attention to his environment. If you are expecting a guest then you hear every car door that slams. If you are an ornithologist you hear each new bird song. If you are in love then you are aware of all stimuli that can be related, even tenuously, to your lover; and if you are feeling thoroughly 'got at' then every hostile nuance in the conversation of those around seems to be significant and personal. It is interesting to remember that last example when confronted by someone who is described as having paranoid ideas. Might it be that, in a social world which contains both hostility and tolerance, he is responding to events or comments which have not warranted your attention and you are perceiving the same world in a more positive and friendly way?

Summary

These comments on perception have been made because this is a particularly significant topic within psychiatry. Hallucinations are only one example of perceptual disorder. Equally important to the therapist are disturbances of body image, experiences of depersonalisation and derealisation and problems arising from faulty interpersonal perception. The topic of interpersonal perception, which includes the formation of impressions, the interpretation of mood and behaviour and the attitudes adopted by individuals within relationships, is a theme which runs through almost every chapter which follows. Cook (1979) sums up its significance: 'The way people see each other determines the way they behave towards each other, so the study of 'person perception' is one of the keys to understanding social behaviour.'

Perception as a cognitive process and perception as a social influence have both been referred to within this section. Unless you are a purist, in terms of psychological research into observable behaviour, it is permissible and useful to combine these perspectives in terms of mental illness. They are interlinked and complementary within any individual's attempt to make sense of his world.

Disturbance of thinking

It is not easy to separate thought and speech. One could say that thought is the process and speech the product through which thinking is expressed. However, it is difficult to rule out the possibility that the way people think is deeply influenced by their vocabulary and verbal ability. When people are unhappy or disturbed we realise their distress through the content of their speech and so, for simplicity, the two will be regarded here as a single dimension.

In order to think effectively an individual needs to know who he is, in what context he is operating and what he hopes to achieve. He needs to be able to refer to past learning and experiences to maintain concentration over a period of time and to interpret the environment and the responses of others. He needs to organise all of this information, to handle abstract as well as concrete concepts, to form hypotheses, to reason the possibilities and probabilities involved and to express this entire process in the signs and symbols which make up language.

Cognition, or thinking, is therefore a very complex process which is reliant on not only intelligence but also on features which include perception, memory, attention, attitudes, concentration, creativity, reasoning and language. At every stage the process is vulnerable to disruption for a number of different reasons. Physical factors include altered consciousness, toxic states induced by metabolic disorder, deficiency, drugs or alcohol, and brain damage or deterioration. Emotional factors include debilitating anxiety, the blocking of information through the use of defence mechanisms, retardation due to depression, shock and fear. Social factors include immaturity, helplessness acquired through learning, features of socialisation, conflict, and other environmental influences. Whatever the reasons, disorders in thinking involve the following wide spectrum.

Consciousness

To be conscious is to know about oneself and about the world. This involves first of all being wakeful, secondly being lucid (that is able to relate clearly to the immediate environment) and thirdly being aware of oneself as a unique and enduring being against a background which includes reality, experience and time.

Wakefulness is essentially a function of the reticular formation, the hypothalamus and frontal lobes. Being essentially a state controlled by the mid-brain it can be affected by physical phenomena such as toxicity or brain damage. It is normally subject to fluctuations as each individual has patterns of sleeping and waking and of activity and non-activity. It is subject to the general state of an individual's physical health and can be disrupted by emotional experiences as different from one another as terror and boredom. Information about wakefulness can be gained not only from overt physical signs such as eye movements and muscle tone but also from electroencephalograms which measure the amount of cerebral electrical activity taking place.

Lucidity involves being able to make use of one's own perceptive, cognitive, intellectual and sensory functions. The degree of lucidity is, of course, closely connected to the degree of wakefulness but involves understanding the environment as well as being aware of it. Information about lucidity is gained by questioning the patient about where he is, what he is doing and why he is doing it.

When problems related to consciousness occur they are usually due to some temporary or permanent damage to the brain. Clouding of consciousness, drowsiness, confusion and delirium, for example, are all problems which are associated with organic conditions.

At the other end of the scale certain patients may describe states of heightened consciousness. Their understanding of the world

seems to be intensely enriched and they report vivid sensory awareness and inspired thinking and feeling. Again, the reasons for these
experiences are normally physiological, typically through taking
stimulant or hallucinogenic drugs. A similar experience of general
stimulation may be reported by patients who are described as
suffering from 'mania' where the aetiology is less clear.

Memory

Memory is a complex process and is well documented within most
basic psychology courses. Memory is the essential component of all
perception, learning and reasoning. It also has a strong affective
component which can be demonstrated by observing how motivation, stress or repugnance can influence forgetting.

An individual's biography, social identity, ability to deal with the
present and capacity to have valid ambitions for the future are all
invested in memory. Any damage to the ability to retain and recall
information is therefore deeply threatening to a person and may
give rise to secondary problems of denial, confabulation or
emotional distress. Psychologists have distinguished between long
and short term memory; both these functions can be disturbed.

Organic factors leading to disturbance of memory can be
recognised in the 'brain failure' of some elderly people and in those
where the brain has been damaged by trauma or by toxic substances
such as alcohol. The nature of the disturbance is related to the
extent of the damage or deterioration but is often associated with
the recall of recent information.

A sudden shock, such as a bang on the head, electro-convulsive
treatment or an intense emotional experience may interfere with the
processing and retention of recent information leading to a memory
gap. The period of time which is 'lost' in this way will vary with
the severity of the shock.

Emotional elements in the maintenance of an effective memory
are more difficult to explain. The phenomenon of total amnesia,
which may be hysterical in origin, or may be a response to an
unbearable degree of stress, is one extreme. Those patients who are
depressed or anxious often complain of having a poor memory; they
find difficulty in retaining both important and trivial details.
Although it may be tempting to ascribe this problem to low levels
of concentration and motivation, this does not really account for the
degree of difficulty that such people are experiencing.

Thinking

This is an artificially broad heading since it could be taken as embracing all of cognition. The word is used here to mean the ability to examine information and to respond to it in an organised way. Thinking involves being able to use the symbols of language and speech coherently. To communicate our thinking to others we need to have symbols and a perception of reality in common with them. Disturbance of thinking can be recognised in a wide variety of disorders. Emotional disturbance can affect the speed of thought, depression of mood often leading to slowness and to difficulty in grasping new information. This should not be confused with a change in pace which is normal in old age and does not necessarily affect the quality of reasoning. In more acute conditions there may be difficulties in thinking clearly at all and the patient complains of blocks and breaks occurring in a train of thought or he may get stuck in a loop of repetitive and unproductive ideas. Melancholy brooding as well as apparently psychotic perseveration may demonstrate this sort of problem.

A lack of control in thinking may also be described by a patient or be observed from the content of his speech. A simple example of this is the 'flight of ideas' which arises from acceleration of thought to the extent that new material intervenes in the expression of every sequence, and superficial associations are formed. Other people complain that ideas are being imposed upon them from outside or are being withdrawn. This latter experience is very close to delusion.

Other disorders of thought involve degrees of apparent irrelevance or incoherence. It is difficult to assess how much of the difficulty lies in the processing of ideas and how much in expressive problems. What comes out may not sound either clear or logical but we can only guess from a person's speech, and from any indication of distress or frustration which accompanies this speech, the degree of disorganisation in his actual thinking.

Delusion

A delusion is a private, firmly held, and personally significant belief about the world. To this extent we may all claim to have a few. The textbooks tell us that a delusion becomes a psychiatric symptom when the beliefs encompassed within it are false. To say that something is false or untrue means that it is incompatible with reality as it is experienced and expressed by those of us who are not deluded. This is not a heretical attempt to obscure the issue, merely a warning that truth is relative. Those people who have disabling delusional beliefs find themselves isolated and alienated from the everyday experiences of other people. They may spend much time brooding over these ideas and may construe unrelated events as providing proof or evidence; in this way systems of delusional ideas are built up.

For some people the social world revolves around their own delusions. A central idea that they are an extraordinary or historically significant person colours all their relationships and perceptions. Others may be able to sustain delusional beliefs alongside an appreciation of the world as perceived by others, or may have isolated delusions which refer only to specific topics or situations. Delusions are not experienced only by those who are described as being psychotic, they are merely an extreme form of unshared belief which may arise from any form of emotional or physical isolation.

Disturbance of mood

It is easier for many of us to understand varieties in mood than to relate to disturbances in perception and cognition. Perhaps this is because we assume our own perceptions and thoughts to be similar to those of other people, whereas we know that our feelings fluctuate, are unpredictable to others and are, to ourselves, unique. We also know from experience that the running of many occupational therapy departments is subject to at least half a dozen uncoordinated menstrual cycles. It is acceptable, and sometimes comforting, to believe that one's mood is affected by physical factors such as physiological needs and the balance or imbalance of hormones. Any suggestion that our perceptions of the world and the way in which we think are subject to such arbitrary influences is curiously more threatening.

Patients who are experiencing difficulties associated with mood may be able to count on a greater degree of empathy from their therapists, but the relationship is still problematic. It is sometimes difficult to know what to say to someone whose misery or inappropriate reaction exceeds our own imagined response to a situation.

There are four major styles of affective disturbance which inhibit communication and relationship. These are lability and rapid fluctuation in mood, inappropriate emotional responses, misery and euphoria.

Emotional lability is typified by immediate reaction to every stimulus. The instantaneous way in which such reactions are produced make them appear superficial, and sometimes irrelevant. The mood invoked is often short lived which leaves one, perhaps unfairly, questioning the validity of the emotions expressed. This style of emotional response is associated with immaturity, intellectual impairment and damage to the brain.

Inappropriate responses are those in which a topic or situation which would normally evoke one set of feelings gives rise to different and incompatible reactions. This is not an entirely abnormal phenomenon as any student, who has answered a classroom question wrongly and collapsed into a heap of giggling mirth, will know. The classic examples of inappropriate affect involve psychotic patients who receive bad news, for example of family bereavement, with apparent amusement. It is not uncommon, however, to find apparently normal people who cannot discuss traumatic periods within their own lives without smiling or laughing in an incongruous way. It is difficult to assess the extent to which such incongruity is the product of embarrassment or defensiveness, and to what extent the emotion felt is truly out of context with the circumstances. Just as thinking and language are difficult to separate, genuine feelings and expressed emotions may not complement each other. It is rarely effective to be impatient with those who find it difficult to represent their feelings accurately, nor is it relevant to determine what a person *should* feel within any set of circumstances. The decision as to whether to confront a person with his own inappropriate reaction, or to accept whatever emotional reacticn he chooses to present, can only be made on an individual basis and in the light of knowledge about other treatment he may be receiving.

Misery is common enough as one of the main features of depressive illness. Extreme unhappiness and negative self-concept frequently occur in other disorders, even when they have not been identified as a major problem. Very few people who are in receipt of psychiatric treatment are consistently happy. Normal fluctuations in mood and fortune include periods of misery but, as sufferers, we retain the knowledge that most subjective experiences are short lived. We know that things will get better, that we will not always feel so foul. Real misery is experienced when one loses touch with the fluid and cyclical nature of existence and comes to believe that there will be no forseeable change. It is a short step then to believing oneself undeserving of improved fortune and responsible for the surrounding waste and sadness. To be told to cheer up can contribute merely another ounce of guilt to the burden. It is difficult for a therapist, a nurse or a relative, to know how to cope with misery as expressed through tears and self-derogatory statements. We know enough to avoid denying them, which is to impede the formation of any relationship, or to reinforce them with the style of sympathy which encourages dependency and helplessness.

The patient who is euphoric or 'high' creates a variation on this problem for himself and for those around him. Extravagant behaviour may be exhilerating, embarrassing or dangerous. It is also exhausting for all concerned. Contrary to superficial descriptions, being high is not the opposite of feeling low. Both are expressions of isolation, both may have physiological antecedents or consequences. As with every other manifestation of psychological distress the causes may be various but the outcome is social disruption.

REFERENCES

Arietie S, Bemporad J 1980 Severe and mild depression, the psychotherapeutic approach. Tavistock, London
Bandura A 1960 Relationship of family patterns to child behaviour disorders. Stanford University Press, Stanford
Cook M 1979 Perceiving others. Methuen, London
Coulter J 1973 Approaches to insanity. Martin Robertson, London
Davison C G, Neale J M 1982 Abnormal psychology, 3rd edn. John Wiley, New York
Maher B A 1966 Principles of psychopathology: an experimental approach. McGraw-Hill, New York
Perls F, Hefferline R F, Goodman P 1951 Gestalt therapy. Penguin Books, Harmondsworth
Scharfetter C 1980 General psychopathology. Cambridge University Press, Cambridge

RECOMMENDED READING

Clare A 1976 Psychiatry in dissent, 2nd edn. Tavistock, London
Cohen J, Clark J H 1979 Medicine, mind and man. W H Freeman, Reading
Croyden-Smith A 1982 Schizophrenia and madness. George Allen and Unwin, London
Curren D, Partridge M, Storey P 1980 Psychological medicine, an introduction to psychiatry. Churchill Livingstone, Edinburgh
Goldberg D, Huxley P 1980 Mental illness in the community. Tavistock, London

Stress and the vulnerable personality

INTRODUCTION

We are all vulnerable personalities, some more so than others, and more so at some times than at others. Most men and women experience stress at some stage. Stress will not be an unexpected result on a morning when the alarm clock has failed to go off, when I have toothache and premenstrual tension, when the car will not start and my husband has already left with a colleague. The tension may well be released by a good kick at the cat which trips me up, or by swearing at traffic lights which are at red. There are days when one can cope with minor setbacks such as these, but on other days the least problem can produce a feeling of stress.

Why is it that perceptions of stress and threats to our own identities differ from one person to another? A patient in hospital who is arriving for treatment for the first time can feel under threat, as can the new student who is uncertain of her role. What is this stress? Why are there variations in vulnerability?

This chapter will discuss the positive and negative aspects of stress, what causes it and how people normally cope. It will also look at the causes of abnormal stress and its effects. Five brief sketches in words will describe some of the more vulnerable amongst us and present some of the solutions available from professional and non-professional sources.

WHAT IS STRESS?

Stress is a common experience but one that is hard to define in specific terms. Many other words such as anxiety and tension seem to be interchangeable. The word stress originates from the physical sciences and means a 'constraining or impelling force' (Concise Oxford Dictionary), and 'effort' or a 'demand upon energy'. In this sense stresses on structures have an optimum point when tension is maintained and breaking point is withheld. Too much stress and the wires will snap.

Tension in human terms suggests a feeling of discomfort and may be described as nervous tension. Tension and anxiety are dependent on each other, although the actual cause of the anxiety may be unconscious. So anxiety, tension and stress are different yet have come to be regarded as synonymous in everyday language. Therefore, in this chapter stress is considered in its widest sense.

Stress as a positive force

Just as tension has an optimal level in mechanical terms so has stress. Many people thrive on stress. At the optimal level for each individual it can be valuable. It keeps us on our toes, sparks off energy and produces the drive to achieve full potential. Without that specific and individual quota of stress some people function below par and can be slow and apathetic. How often are assignments finally completed at the last minute? For many, without that pressure which is brought about by limited time, there is insufficient motivation to harness thoughts and organise words into acceptable scripts. As with the writer facing an empty page so does the climber approaching a new pitch feel muscles tense ready for action and feel the senses alert to all eventualities, while judgement is sharpened and decisions are made. Sometimes the monotony of everyday life causes individuals to seek shortlived yet stressful situations in order to test out those senses, to produce excitement and exhilaration and the feeling of power and achievement. But these stresses which are sought for, are generally within the control of the individual, whether gambling, scrambling or vandalising. The successful outcomes of such situations provide the individual with, or reinforce for him, a clearer concept of his own ability to survive, as well as providing an enjoyable experience, even if this is sometimes in retrospect.

Stress as an unpleasant experience

Stress is inevitable and for some may be a vital part of their experience with each new event providing new challenges. For others, life's many and varied events bring their own stress and strain. Changing circumstances like one's first day at school bring exposure to new people, new systems of organisation, written and unwritten rules and the law of the jungle. All this and more can be rather intimidating until one learns to cope and finds ways of ensuring survival. Taking examinations, the storms of adolescence, one's first job, leaving home, marriage, responsibility for children, illness, retirement and bereavement all produce different levels of stress for each person, according to the individual's thresholds and how each perceives the world.

Many joys may be associated with childbirth but the very fact that it is a new experience brings uncertainties and anxieties. What if the baby cries? Can I cope? Most parents do cope but when the crying continues without the baby responding to comforting, feeding, changing or being played with, when the intensity and duration increases beyond understanding, then stress for the parent becomes unpleasant. Depending on the personality of the parent and on other stresses which might be present at the time, behaviour will be affected. Perhaps, help will be sought. On the other hand, the baby might be left to cry out of earshot or, worse, become victim of child abuse.

Stress can be unpleasant and can originate from both external and internal factors. The external factors are those in the environment and their effects depend on how they are perceived by the individual. Is it friendly and supportive or hostile and demanding? Internal factors relate to either physical or psychological aspects of the individual. When one is tired, suffering from premenstrual tension or from a specific illness, the baby's crying is much more likely to cause stress than at other times when thresholds are not lowered. Also, there is the fact that susceptibility to anxiety can be a personality trait and this, accompanied by such things as motivation, cognitive skills and ability to assert oneself, can affect the level of stress experienced and the response made.

When different stages in life are analysed for common stressful factors it would seem that a generalisation can be made that acute stress occurs when there is a threat to one's identity or integrity, when there has been a change in status with a resulting change in role and before one's adaptive behaviour has yet been established. Temporarily, at least, the individual is not in control and lack of control leads to anxiety. If the stress is likely to be short-lived then the alerted senses will assist in dealing with the situation and control will be regained. However, if the stress is excessive in terms of duration or intensity, and if no apparent changes in behaviour alleviate it, then energy and drive will be sapped and motivation to continue seeking alternative behaviours, which will enable one to cope successfully, will be undermined.

Take, for example, the new patient's arrival in the occupational therapy department for the first time. The environment looks unfamiliar and, unless there has been thorough preparation before arrival, it may resemble a torture chamber with overhead beams, slings and adapted equipment, or look like a very busy workshop. Temporarily, at least, the secure role of being a patient in the ward has been lost and adjustment has not yet been made to the role expected during treatment. This may seem an exaggeration, but it illustrates the point that there is a whole continuum of stress associated with changing roles. At one end of the scale, there is the relatively easy change from that of patient to participant in a programme of treatment. While at the other end, due to, say, chronic illness there are irrevocable changes of role and established patterns of life, with consequent loss of security. Thus, in one dimension there can be gradations of causative factors related to the environment and in other dimension there are variations in personality leading to a greater or lesser ability to cope.

Physical symptoms of stress and resulting behaviour

Continual exposure to stress beyond individual thresholds has distressing physical concomitants, such as increased heart beat, sweating and irregular breathing. However, man's ability to anticipate and to reason can reduce anxiety levels depending on previous experience, learning and personality. Equally, of course, these same factors can induce it. This is described more fully in Chapter 8.

We are all aware of the internal physical signs of stress and may well continue with our everyday lives regardless. But there comes a breaking point when stress is manifested externally. It may show itself in short-lived irritation with whom or whatsoever comes along first, in either a frustration-releasing expletive or a more lengthy outburst and argument. Interpersonal clashes often result when personal control is reduced, and there is also a predisposition to accidents when under stress. The individual may be less alert to surroundings, be preoccupied or misinterpret the warning signals and so fail to avoid a collision.

HOW DO PEOPLE COPE?

Strategies for coping

Already, some behaviours such as swearing have been referred to. These will draw on the 'fight' mechanism of the sympathetic nervous system and may give immediate release of tension in the short-term, but long-term results may produce further complications and stress—for example, hitting the traffic warden instead of the parking meter. When aware of stress building up, and recognising tension in muscles, the wise will seek to change their behaviour. Temporary avoidance of the stressful situation by escaping to the cinema or for a holiday abroad works for some while others will work off tension and energy through sport or digging the garden. Deep breathing exercises and relaxing, having a nice cup of tea or a smoke can also help reduce tension. Of course, these can be done in the company of others and many cope with stress through a supportive network of family or friends. These may help one either to confront the causes and find the solutions to the stress, or alternatively to escape from it through agreeable social activity.

Stress in all its forms is coped with better by some than others. We all have our own individual strengths and strategies, whether they are sleep, sex or sedatives. The following is a practical example of a useful strategy. Given numerous demands and pressure of work, there can be a fear of losing control. However, a deliberate withdrawal to write down and arrange in order of priority all the tasks awaiting to be done, can help restore control. But whatever the cause of the stress, personal maturity with a positive and imaginative approach is required to help find a balance between work and play and to introduce progressively differentiated responses, adaptive behaviour and new strategies for coping.

Fortunately for us, our ability to learn new patterns of behaviour and to coordinate actions unconsciously means that situations which once produced stress, such as coping with school or learning to drive a car, can be done with comparatively little effort. Thus, while there is no denying the existence of stress, it is accepted that as we become familiar with a situation, our adaptive behaviour becomes progressively more automatic and that, having learnt to cope successfully with one situation, we are then ready to meet the next potentially stressful problem.

Unconscious mechanisms for coping with stress

Stress, tension, anxiety—these diffuse emotional states with accompanying physical effects can be painful unless preventative measures are taken to control them. Besides conscious strategies as briefly described above, the subconscious mind also makes use of unconscious mechanisms. These are attempts by the ego to reduce anxiety and threats to the individual's self-esteem. The number of defence mechanisms and their differentiation is controversial but the following descriptions of rationalisation, projection, repression, and sublimation serve as examples of unconscious mechanisms for coping with stress.

Rationalisation takes place when the blame for failure is shifted onto something else. 'A poor workman blames his tools.' 'There are not enough staff to treat everyone properly.' These are not necessarily 'true' or 'rational' excuses but they make us feel better and help to justify conduct so that behaviour is excused.

Projection, as the word suggest, means attributing to another a weakness within oneself. We all have undesirable traits, but it can be painful to admit or even to acknowledge them openly. Hence, a mean person may well claim that his meanness is solely in response to that of others; or 'everyone is so unfriendly, I'm always on my own!'

Memories and facts which are painful for the individual may be removed from conscious awareness and become repressed. Repression is not intentional, as would be the case if something was 'suppressed'. At one end of the scale a dental appointment might be repressed and forgotten until too late, while at the other, repressed memories of name, address, job would lead to a state of amnesia. It is not that they have been completely forgotten for they can become accessible under certain circumstances, but that they would produce feelings of anxiety or guilt if brought back into conscious awareness. Hence, repression can protect the individual.

Sublimation is perhaps one of the most successful defence mechanisms for it channels unacceptable motives into socially acceptable behaviour. Aggressive outlets may be found in sporting activities; a subconscious desire to have a child may direct this instinctive energy into caring for others and so remove possible frustration and tension.

ABNORMAL STRESS

This section will consider the cause and effect of stress which has become intolerable, leading to maladaptive behaviour and 'psychiatric illness'. As outlined above we are all exposed to stress. Sometimes it is to our benefit; sometimes it is painful. The results will depend largely on our personalities, previous experiences, social support and behaviour. Let us now consider what it is about some personalities which makes them more vulnerable.

Personality

The development of personality has long fascinated philosophers, psychologists and others and many different classifications have been described, but it is easier to define different types than to account for the differences. However, the simple teachings of Hippocrates and of Galen did link body chemistry to emotion, and we know that excessive anxiety can lead to ulcers, loss of weight and increased activity of bowel and bladder. Hippocrates (5 BC) taught that the human body was composed of four elements: air, water, fire and earth. Galen (2 AD) said that these elements corresponded to substances in the body: blood, phlegm, yellow and black bile; and, depending on the quantity of each within each individual, so did the personality differ, of which four categories were identifiable: sanguine, phlegmatic, choleric and melancholic. However, since there are many different characteristics by which individual personalities can be judged, and since moods can vary, it is extremely difficult to categorise people subjectively into only four types. Yet to have a framework of personality types does lead the therapist towards a better understanding of the individual. C. J. Jung (1875–1961) and H. J. Eysenck (1916–) have added the dimensions of introversion–extroversion and stable–unstable

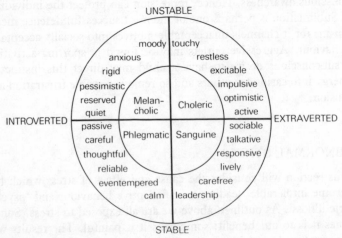

Fig. 2.1 Modified from Eysenck and Rachman (1970)

respectively, along which lines a much greater range of traits can be identified. If, in fact, both ancient and modern theories are combined we get a schematic diagram allowing for much greater variation and understanding.

Objective methods for classifying people, i.e. personality inventories and factor analysis, have often been criticised as being unreliable, but there is increasing evidence of their usefulness. Take for example the Depression Scale in the Minnesota Multiple Personality Inventory (MMPI); this will identify not only those individuals who are sick enough to need psychiatric attention but also those whose depression is hidden from casual observation and is called 'masked' or 'smiling depression'. These subjects score high on those parts of the inventory which reveal their feelings of uselessness, pessimism, lack of self-confidence, tendency to worry and introversion (Hathaway & McKinley, 1951). Depression may become a personality trait. Some will claim that personality develops so early on in life that it can almost be considered innate. Others such as Levett (1968) say that a particular emotional state, for example anxiety, will play a part in the development of personality through its influence on behaviour, the outcome of which will influence how the person perceives himself and his behaviour in the future. The development of personality is therefore a dynamic affair.

Effects of learning

The anxious person is one who is frightened of being hurt and of being unable to cope. This fear may be a conditioned response resulting from a frightening experience. Take for example the famous experiment by Watson (1920) when young Albert was shown a white rat. He showed no fear of it until its presence was accompanied by a frightening noise. Thereafter, he became afraid of the rat and of many other white furry objects. Albert's fear, like many other irrational fears, was learnt through association with a rationally frightening stimulus. If the person is unable to escape from the frightening, painful or stressful stimulus, despite many efforts, then he becomes helpless and passive. If, however, under previously stressful circumstances initiative and action have enabled escape then the person will respond actively again. 'What gets learnt when the environment is controllable, or is uncontrollable, has profound consequences for the entire repertoire of behaviour.' (Seligman, 1975). Helplessness can therefore be learned and, just as Albert's fear was transferred to other furry objects, so can helplessness, acquired under traumatic circumstances, be transferred to other situations. Thus, the individual begins to fail to discriminate between those circumstances when he is truly helpless and those in which he can take control. The spoilt child can become helpless and passive, never needing to work or to fight for what he wants. The 'victim' of the welfare state who is denied his sense of responsibility in making decisions, and having some control over his own life, loses the motivation to compete. He becomes apathetic and lazy. As long as one of our alcoholic patients, Nick, was sleeping under an upturned boat and working hard to survive each day, he retained a sense of purpose and well-being. As soon as a hostel roof was provided for him with regular meals at times set by the establishment he lost his identity and returned to the bottle. From this it is easy to see how institutional helplessness can develop and chronic conditions arise unless active steps are take to mitigate against it.

A simulation game used in teacher training (Thatcher, 1980) imposes contrived handicaps, such as restricted vision, hearing or movement, on each participant. They are then asked to carry out a number of simple tasks such as wiring a plug or answering written questions. The instructions are incomplete or incomprehensible; the equipment is broken and the 'teacher' constantly criticises those who are slow or incompetent. Imagine how you might feel, or better still try it out. After this training exercise, to increase their own sensitivity to those less competent than themselves, participants examine the experience and how they responded during the active phase of the exercise. The results of consistent experience as emulated in this game can produce a cognitive set which says 'I'm a failure'. Thereafter behaviour is almost self-fulfilling. The person who sees himself as a failure and does not have protective defence mechanisms, fails to set targets, or sets them too high, or has unrealistic standards and therefore fails ever to achieve his own expectations. This sense of failure is often reinforced by the family and friends whose well meaning advice 'you shouldn't be such a worrier' does nothing to change the individual's concept of himself. Invariably there are some children who in school are picked out by classmates and teachers as being the shy, silly and stupid ones. They fail in a variety of social situations and come to think of themselves as hopeless failures. On the other hand, children who are spoilt, or who are constantly told how wonderful they are and seem to succeed in everything, may have a disastrous reaction to their first experience of failure if they have never been faced with such a problem before. The child needs to learn from an early age to cope with hurtful responses from others and from painful emotions. People who have learnt to cope successfully with the bully, the angry parent, disappointment and jealousy will have a greater repertoire for coping with other situations in the future. The course that does not really stretch students, and is too easy, will make them devalue themselves, develop a sense of apathy, and fail to prepare them for future challenges.

Traumatic experiences

Personality and early experiences can produce stress and lead to the development of an anxious personality. Stress can also be caused by environmental pressures and traumatic experiences.

It is easy to see why urban stress with unemployment, noise, overcrowding and poverty can make people feel bad about their circumstances and then about themselves, but it is difficult to show direct links between these factors alone and psychiatric illness. Although some may suffer, others seem to thrive. The situation is very complex for there are many variables affecting behaviour. Similarly, traumatic experiences of rape, war, isolation, illness and bereavement can become pathological for some.

Deprivation and death

Deprivation and death of a loved one can be extremely traumatic and a number of studies have added to our understanding. Deprivation can be experienced in different ways. Spitz reported in the early 1940s on infants who were cared for in an institution which provided basic necessities such as food and clean clothing but the minimum of physical contact and social stimulation. Regular meals, cleanliness and a cot to oneself were found to be insufficient for healthy development. These children put on little weight and some died for no other apparent reason than lack of mothering. This is an extreme case but it helps us to appreciate the extent of the emotional deprivation in psychoneurotic patients who attempt suicide, compared with a related group who do not (Walton, 1958; Bruhn, 1962). Earle and Earle (1961), instead of comparing groups of patients as in the previous studies, matched individuals who had lost one or both parents in childhood, with those who had not. While results showed no significant increase in psychiatric diagnosis there was a tendency towards broken marriage, poor work record and crime. Thus parental loss may at the very least, contribute towards instability of the personality but this loss may have been precipitated by unhappiness and other domestic problems. However, when loss is due to early parental death, then this factor has been shown to be excessive in psychiatric patients. A significant number of patients compared with 500 controls had lost a parent through death before they were ten (Birtchnell, 1970). He also showed that an excessive number of patients had experienced recent death of a parent, i.e. between 1–5 years prior to their first admission; and that early or recent parental death was particularly high amongst severly depressed patients who attempted suicide.

Bereavement is usually followed by three stages of grief; sudden shock and disbelief, followed by acceptance and grieving, with subsequent adjustment to a different life-style. Since the years following bereavement represent a period of instability and adjustment it is not surprising to find that many psychiatric patients have recently experienced the death of a close person.

Relationships

People often seek out the company of others who reinforce the concepts they have of themselves. But sometimes the individual finds himself in the situation where messages seems to contradict themselves and he becomes confused as to how the other person sees him. For example, the child who is given all sorts of material benefits—toys and clothes—yet is constantly told: 'Go away and play', 'Don't bother me,' may believe himself to be loved, and at the same time feel himself rejected.

Sometimes people find themselves in a 'double-bind' situation where it does not matter how they respond; which ever way, they will be punished. Take for example the teenager who returns late only to be told: 'I'm glad you're home. I've been worried sick, but you're going to get a beating for being so late.' When such experiences are consistently repeated, insecurity and confusion about one's own identity can arise. 'Does mother really care?'

We all play games to satisfy personal needs. Mature relationships are on an adult to adult level. Immature ones arise when one member adopts either an inappropriate parental or childish role (Berne, 1964). Some marriages for example are based on relationships where the dominant partner can control the other or where one plays the part of victim and the other of rescuer. There could be many reasons why therapists marry their patients besides love. Indeed, there can be many hidden motives why people choose to be therapists. Professional workers are often faced with the dilemma of how much support, advice and friendship should be given and at what point it should be withdrawn and for what reasons. Are they strictly therapeutic or are these subjective personal motives? If these dilemmas and others of an interpersonal nature, whether at work or in the family, remain unresolved, there is a sense of failure, and illness can be engendered. Obviously family relationships and structures affect early experience. Studies have shown that alcoholism is more common in last-born males, and (Rutter et al, 1975) that neurotic disturbances are more frequent in eldest rather than youngest children. It is not surprising to learn that there is a high incidence of physical and psychiatric illness in parents of children referred to child guidance centres (Rutter, 1966). Tension and anxiety within the home are easily transmitted and the sick, stressed behaviour of parents creates insecurity and provides a poor model for children to learn from.

EFFECTS OF VULNERABILITY TO STRESS

Already several references have been made to the effects of stress on people who are not in control of their circumstances, who are less self-disciplined and less comfortable with themselves and others, who are unable to externalise feelings to produce anger or laughter and who lack environmental support. It is very difficult to establish causative links, but psychological problems associated with the above may present themselves in an anxiety state, an obsessive–compulsive disorder, a conversion reaction, depression, phobia, addiction to drugs or alcohol, sexual perversion, suicide, or in a mixture of two or more of these problems, for example, in an anxiety state with depressive features or a hysterical state with anxiety features. Whatever neurotic diagnostic label is given, behaviour in general leads to withdrawal from the threatening, stressful circumstances into a more predictable world, whether through resorting to irrational fears of illness or through the apathy of depression. The neurotic person is often preoccupied with old events and people. The symptomatology and diagnosis will depend to a large extent on the premorbid personality and the characteristics which predominate.

Anxiety state

The term 'anxiety state' tends, unfortunately, to be widely used and has almost become synonymous with 'psyhiatric illness'. 'Normal' anxiety arises when there is a sense of specific or generalised personal danger as during war. Under such circumstances there is agitation, and a heightened responsiveness by the body to act. This anxiety becomes abnormal and pathological when it arises and persists without adequate cause. The degree of anxiety may range from restlessness to an acute panic attack and fear of something dreadful being about to happen. Such anxiety is often called 'free floating'. The patient may be irritable, unable to concentrate, has a poor appetite, sleeps fitfully and gives reports of wild dreams. Physical symptoms cover the whole range of those associated with an increase in output of adrenaline from the automatic nervous system as previously described. The personality often tends towards anxiety either as a result of upbringing or genetic predisposition. The anxious person may have feelings of inferiority and inadequency yet set himself high standards and be ambitious. As a result he takes on more and more and finds it difficult to relax until exhaustion or sudden excessive stress causes him to stop. Without intervention, acute episodes of fear and anxiety can lead to a chronic state. An anxiety state, however, can also be brought on by the removal of life's sustaining stress, for example when a person retires or is faced with sudden unemployment.

Obsessive–compulsive disorder

Some people react to stress with obsessional thoughts and ruminations, compulsive acts or doubts and indecisions. Normal experience includes ritualistic games, daily routines and occasional persistency of a tune in one's head. But when happiness and efficiency are impaired and these rituals, routines and ruminations become time-consuming and disruptive to daily life then we have obsessionalism or an obsessional–compulsive disorder in need of treatment. Pathological obsessions are constant preoccupations with thoughts and feelings, leading often to compulsive acts, which cannot be got rid of by voluntary effort; for example, persistent checking of the gas switch in response to the constant doubt that it has not been turned off. Usually the obsessive-compulsive behaviour arises from a subconscious need to control an underlying fear and to establish some sort of order. The person knows what he is doing yet cannot stop it. He has insight into the irrationality of his behaviour yet is unaware of the underlying motives which are often of a sexual or aggressive nature. compulsive hand-washing several times a day may be a symbolic manifestation of a deeper disturbance. It might be that feelings of guilt have been severely repressed. The compulsive handwashing can be exhausting and the fears of going insane may lead to anxiety or depression. Obsessional personalities are more liable to develop these symptoms than non-obsessional personalities. However, the latter tend to have a better prognosis, especially if the onset of behaviour is related to a particular stress.

Conversion reaction

Stress can produce an hysterical state where underlying psychological problems are converted to physical symptoms and attention becomes focussed on these, thereby reducing the anxiety associated with the problem. The patient may complain of loss of memory, or motor or sensory disturbances such as paralysis of a limb, impaired eyesight, back pain or headaches. Where there is no organic foundation and the complaint carries a personal gain for the patient then it is described as hysteria or, more commonly nowadays, as a conversion reaction. Although the patient may gain from the symptoms of his, or more likely her, physical ailment, the ailment is real to her and she is unaware of the subconscious motives. They have been well repressed. Hysteria is in fact an extreme form of the defence mechanism of repression. Patients with a conversion reaction use their symptoms in such a way that they can dominate their surroundings and so gain control of others. As a result, anxiety is reduced and they escape from the stress-provoking situation. Hysterical symptoms may occur in anyone under sufficient stress but they are more generally seen in those with personality characteristics which are shallow, dramatic, histrionic and immature. The family background may be one that is overprotective and emotional, so patterns of dependency are learnt from an early age. The more a person is predisposed to hysterical behaviour and learns not only that the physical symptoms gain escape from stress but that there are secondary gains of sympathy and attention, the more such behaviour will be elicited. The treatment of a conversion reaction can be difficult unless the immediate cause giving rise to the condition has been overcome. Alas for the persistant hysteric, short-term gains are valued more than gains which might be possible in the long-term if the hysterical behaviour pattern was broken. For some, there might be little attraction in growing-up and taking on adult responsibilities if childish or invalid behaviour keeps one dependent and spoilt. For another, should the ammesia lift, an unhappy marriage or impending exposure for embezzlement may have to be faced. These are only very brief examples but it is worth noting how relatively few patients these days seem to present with dramatic reactions such as sudden paralysis. Instead complaints are more vague and are difficult to distinguish from organic conditions.

Depression

Depression is a very common emotional state and an understandable response to the stress and horror that is reported within society today. Like 'anxiety state', 'depression' tends to be used as a 'umbrella-like' term covering a multitude of possible causes yet prompting a speedy prescription of 'antidepressants'. Depression may be associated directly or indirectly with many different conditions — debilitating physical conditions, Parkinsonism and schizophrenia. It may accompany other neurotic conditions or be full-blown, deep-seated and endogenous. My purpose here is to look at it in its broadest sense as a symptom rather than diagnostic category, for although so common, it is still poorly understood.

The patient in all probability will look depressed with furrowed brow. If he or she smiles at all it will be tense and forced. Movements are slow and sluggish and posture is often stooped as though the weight of the world is on the person's shoulders. He complains of loss of appetite, loss of vitality, loss of interest and of poor concentration. He complains in varying degrees of tiredness yet sleeps poorly. For some, sleep comes readily as though it is a hoped-for panacea, yet the person awakes early. Mood may vary from day to day and from morning to evening but he is generally irritable and anxious, preoccupied with his situation yet ambivalent about action. He is self-deprecating, feels wasted and useless to the point where suicidal thoughts or even attempts have been entertained. This may happen, in particular, when mood improves and volition returns, as though there is a sudden awareness of the depths of the depression just experienced, and a fear of being faced again with such a state of mind.

If the depression has been brought on by a sudden or irreparable loss, such as that of spouse or status, then adjustment may be slow. If, however, it is a reaction to a stress which can be removed, and if the person is not generally melancholic by nature, then prognosis can be good.

Phobias

These may arise in several neurotic conditions—as part of a compulsive disorder, personality disorder or in depression. Phobias are inappropriate fears. Where the fear is related to one specific object it is usually the result of learning, with overgeneralisation and a failure to discriminate in an anxiety-prone person. The fear can be of anything from mice to men, from being shut in or of having cancer. The person recognises the irrationality of his fear which may produce mild anxiety or a panic attack. The physical symptoms experienced in a panic attack may include a few or all of the following: dyspnoea, palpitations, chest pain, choking, dizziness, faintness, trembling, sweating, hot and cold flushes, tingling and feelings of unreality. Little wonder the phobic person seeks to avoid the object of his fear. It can be considerably disruptive to everyday life. Agoraphobia, or fear of public spaces, is perhaps one of the most disruptive. It tends to affect women more than men and is sometimes called the 'housebound housewife' syndrome. Where the fear is directed to something specific rather than the result of deepseated problems, then treatment with relaxation, tranquillisers, hypnosis or systematic desensitisation is usually successful.

Addiction to alcohol and drugs

Addiction may be a symptom of many disorders. Many experiencing stress may seek escape through drink and drugs, the physical effects of which may remove despondency, anxiety and inhibitions, may reduce feelings of gloom and guilt and invoke those of well-being, of being in control and being sociable and likeable. Relief is temporary but the intake may become habitual leading to dependency. It is a sad reflection on society that where there is unemployment, poverty, broken homes and violence, there is a high incidence of alcoholism. It is ironic that the economic aspects of alcoholism merely add more social disasters thus building up a vicious circle and solving few problems. Addiction may also become part of the life-style of those in more favourable circumstances but whose affluence, upbringing and education have left them idle and bored, and defective in their personal development. In order to compensate for feelings of inadequacy and lack of courage to direct their own lives, people take drugs to give themselves a prop. For some it enables them to 'impress' others and to keep in with a peer group, at the same time snubbing society and its values. It is estimated that about half the teenage addicts will be off all drugs within 10–12 years but for others the prognosis is more serious. Some die. Treatment is only successful when an alcoholic or drug addict commits himself to a treatment programme and regime of total abstention.

Sexual problems

On the one hand sexual activity can produce relaxation and reduce stress, but on the other it can create difficulties and frustrations depending on the compatibility and comfort experienced by the couple involved in the relationship. Sexual problems may appear central to unhappiness when in fact they are secondary to other neurotic conditions. Anxiety and obsessional behaviour can interfere with spontaneity, and phobic defences may lead to frigidity and impotence. People seeking counselling often focus on sexual problems when other stressful aspects of the relationship need to be brought out and talked about just as much.

These days there is less prejudice and fewer signs of moral disapproval towards homosexuals, given that they are consenting adults. The desire to have a sexual relationship with someone of the same sex may stem from early childhood experiences whereby stress was associated with someone of the opposite sex. Comfort may be gained through the homosexual relationship but it may also produce severe stress and feelings of guilt and shame, as can also accompany masturbation, fetishism, transvestism, masochism and sadism. These anomalies become disorders when they are antisocial or are destructive of the individual's life. Pleasure may be obtained in the short-term but for some the long-term consequences can include fear of exposure, a distortion or lack of self-esteem, incapacitating guilt and subsequent depression or anxiety.

Suicide and attempted suicide

Suicide is hardly a symptom but a pretty drastic piece of overt behaviour intent on destroying the self and so escaping from stress into oblivion without caring about the outcome. If, however, self-poisoning or rather self-injury is unsuccessful and in fact was never truly serious, then it is often seen as a 'cry for help' and perhaps as an attempt to manipulate significant people. Suicide is high amongst those who are severely depressed and have recently lost a parent, or who lost a parent in childhood. It is also more common amongst those who are single, childless, alcoholic, isolated, unemployed, recently impoverished and who lack religious beliefs. On the basis of the foregoing in this chapter, perhaps you can hypothesise why people in these different social circumstances should have neither internal strengths nor external resources to enable them to cope.

Psychiatric illness in general

Strictly speaking if this were a textbook on psychiatry based on the medical model, the use of the term 'neurosis' would refer solely to the categories of: anxiety states, obsessional–compulsive disorders, phobias and conversion reactions. Each of these contain exaggerated features of behaviour with which normal people can identify. They are exaggerated forms of normal defence mechanisms, exaggerated to the point where they become neurotic symptoms which the individual has learnt to use to defend himself against stress and anxiety and so increase feelings of security. As stress increases so do the efforts at self-protection until they reach maladaptive proportions and fail totally to control the anxiety. Nevertheless, they still establish patterns of behaviour which are later repeated despite their inadequency at restoring a healthy balance. These are exaggerated forms of normal behaviour whereas alcoholism, addiction and sexual problems in medical terminology would come under the heading of personality disorders, and depression would be an affective disorder. In looking at the psychiatric effects of vulnerability, different problems have been briefly described prior to the next section which considers real people freed from medical labels.

VULNERABLE PERSONALITIES

The following case histories serve to illustrate some of the causes and effects of stress in vulnerable personalities.

The first, Paul, shows how poverty of experience can lead to dependency. This form of deprivation gives little opportunity for learning how to take responsibility for oneself, or for having a repertoire of behaviours which will meet familiar and not-so-familiar situations. Thus, there is little self-esteem, and self-perception is largely negative. 'The self is created out of experience of reward and punishment, approbation and disapproval, and parental attitudes are of prime significance in personality development.' (Taulbee & Wright, 1971)

The second, Mary, illustrates how the loss of a 'love-object' can lead to a change in status and role with resulting stress. This person had adopted a narrow perception of the world and herself, despite previous personal strengths, and so had to relearn previous adaptive skills and rebuild her ego-strength in order to cope on her own.

The third, Sheila, also concerns someone who has lost her husband but whose previous personality and experiences are different, as are her emotional responses and present maladaptive defence mechanisms.

The fourth, Jenny, describes a more clear-cut case of stress being shown through compulsive behaviour but one that was initially camouflaged in ambiguous terms of anxiety and depression.

The fifth person, Jim, typifies a depressive reaction in one whose job and marriage fail simultaneously.

Paul

Paul is the only child of elderly parents who have overprotected him. At the age of thirty his father still fastened his coat for him and was holding his hand to and from the treatment centre. Regardless of mutual feelings of affection and physical support, this reinforced his state of dependency. Paul had a life-time of experiencing failure and rejection, from bullying in school to hurtful teasing in the factory where he did a simple routine task. Failure in social relationships and lack of control over his own movements produced stresses which showed themselves through apathy and loss of concentration. He became a hazard at work and was dismissed, with resulting withdrawal from all social contacts into a safer world bounded by earphones and music. On admission to the day hospital he was mute and restless and unable to sit still for more than a few minutes at a time. He was neither psychotic nor defective.

Over a period of about a year he changed dramatically within the safe, friendly environment where praise was given for every accomplishment, from initially saying his name to walking home independently. Through active attention, reassurance, support and encouragement in personal contacts he had become assertive and shows a dry sense of humour. Although still unemployed, he goes out walking on his own and to the cinema. He is also learning to cook with a view to future independence.

Mary

Mary is a very attractive thirty-seven year old. She trained as a nursery nurse but for 14 years lived with a man by whom she had a longed-for child. Her common-law husband was a weak person and a gambler who spent her savings, destroyed outside friendships and had spells in prison. Throughout, she disregarded other important aspects of life such as her own identity and other personal needs. But despite his shortcomings she stuck by him, supporting and loving him till one day he suddenly went off without any explanation, with a young neighbour. Mary's world collapsed. She was lonely, lost and confused without John. It could be suggested that she had been playing a parental role to both her daughter and to John, to the point where John rebelled and escaped from being dependent on her. But this was a role she was particularly good at. However, it was inappropriate for coping with mature adult relationships. Mary became tearful and withdrawn, full of doubts and a sense of failure.

Treatment centred on helping her come to terms with her loss, reinforcing the many qualities she has, and taking control of her own life. It was also important for her to relearn how to relate to others on an adult, as opposed to parental, level. The attitudes of staff were passive and friendly, waiting for Mary to take the initiative to examine the cause of her stress, thus avoiding making her dependent on them for decisions affecting her life. Within a year she developed some insight to her own unconscious needs, took an allotment, started a catering course and is enjoying a social life.

Sheila

Sheila is in her sixties. Her husband died of a heart attack four years ago and she is ridden with guilt, in the belief that had she called an ambulance herself instead of waiting for the health centre to contact their G.P., he might not have died. As a nurse, she had recognised the signs of a heart attack but, as the product of a Victorian, middle class upbringing, she had to wait for the authority of the doctor rather than act independently. Now she is unable to cope with the guilt plus the loss of her husband. The problem is compounded by decreasing mobility due to arthritis, and by conflict between her twenty-year-old daughter's morality and her own religious beliefs. Throughout life she has been dependent on others for making important decisions—on nanny, parent, boarding school staff and then her husband. However, she was a competent Sister in starched collar. Now she tries to cope by being that busy competent person doing things for others so that she never has time to examine her own emotions or those of her daughter. For four years she has been avoiding help because it is too painful. Now that she is physically less mobile and has to be at home more, all the guilt and feelings of helplessness surface, resulting in indecisiveness, distress and depression.

Staff in the treatment centre which she attends daily are giving practical support in order to sort out her husband's affairs, and are helping her to accept changing attitudes in society and thus accept her daughter's behaviour. She is also learning that she cannot be running around after others and making assumptions about what they might think or want, for she is then only running away from herself. Treatment may take time while Sheila learns to accept a different life style, in all probability on her own. Staff are firm but kind and other patients confront her about her over-motherliness.

Jenny

Jenny is a small, lively and youthful fifty-year-old. She laughs at the world and it laughs at her, or so it seems. Her tough and alcoholic lorry-driving husband has left her after thirty years. She admits to being frightened on her own, leaves a light on at night and has a hammer by her bed—not common behaviour perhaps, but not irrational under the circumstances. She says that she is depressed and lonely and that she has lost her friends. There was little evidence, when participating in the group's activities, to substantiate this until the day when everyone else was joining in a session on relaxation and she opted to remain sitting on the chair rather than lie on the floor. 'The floor is dirty you see, even the chair is dirty and as soon as I get home everything, even my hair, would have to be washed, because I feel dirty.' In fact this, and even more obsessional behaviour, involving washing and rewashing clothes, had been going on for more than twenty years. Although the family knew, it was a taboo subject lest outsiders though her mad. At last, having admitted to this abnormal covert behaviour to the group, they helped her examine when and why she first began to feel dirty. Through honesty and openness with the group, she learnt that she was still accepted and not rejected as mad, but rather valued for herself and her humour. Her self-esteem rose and a behavioural programme was drawn up between her and the psychologist which helped reduce the compulsive, disruptive behaviour.

Jim

Jim was a happy-go-lucky chap. His marriage over the past 13 years had been happy. Work as an engineer was good for there was plenty to be done and the money, along with his wife's earnings, enabled them to have a nice home and three holidays abroad each year. There were threats of redundancies but he had changed jobs in the past and found another easily. And anyway he had already survived three cuts in this present firm and was ready to meet the demands being made on maintenance staff in order to keep abreast of the new technology in electronics. He had been to the States on a course. They would not want to lose him. But they did—three weeks after the course. As for his wife, her desire for a stimulating career, and an unexpected change from a bank to a multinational industry, led to a jet setting life style and a change in her priorities. She could not be at home for a celebratory wedding anniversary meal. She would leave suddenly on business trips. One day she announced she was leaving Jim, packed her bags and went. A week later he was made redundant. His life collapsed. For days he kept the curtains closed so he would not be seen or disturbed. He crept out in the evening to a corner shop to get groceries. He did not want to meet neighbours and they left him alone. He felt ashamed and a failure. Brandy and overdose, locked car in a locked garage would end it. But his son found him on a casual visit. Lucky for him his 'cry for help' was heard and he was referred to the day hospital.

Now, a year later, when he recalls the feelings of that time he says he felt, 'a sense of nothingness. I did not want, I could not do, anything. I was useless and wasted. I had lost all confidence and no one wanted me'.

Undemanding support from staff and fellow patients gradually gave way to Jim being asked to do simple tasks such as replacing a light bulb. Gradually confidence returned and he took on voluntary work, making aids and equipment in the occupational therapy department of a general hospital. Enjoyment of this environment and alleviation of his depressive state led to full employment in the hospital. The divorce is through; he has a flat of his own and is appreciating and contributing to the humanitarian aspects of his new role of working with people rather than machines.

Unlike some of the others described here, Jim has an apparently strong and adequate personality. He has been made vulnerable temporarily by the circumstances of his life, but has been able to use past experiences of success in order to adapt to a new life style. However, the acuteness of his distress and vulnerability during the time when he was ill is unquestionable.

ADVANTAGES AND DISADVANTAGES OF PROFESSIONAL INTERVENTION

For those more vulnerable personalities whose stresses have become intolerable and for whom there is no easy or immediate solution, the search for the cause, and the initiation of solutions, must be sought through others. Theories and treatments are described in other chapters but it is also important to evaluate the effectiveness or otherwise of professional intervention. This final section will consider some of the advantages and disadvantages, as well as the dynamics, of a therapeutic setting.

The first problem can arise when a patient first reports to his general pactitioner with an underlying problem of stress. Often the GP's lack of time, coupled with the patient's ignorance of his feelings or his resistence to exposing the real discomforts of guilt, jealousy or 'don't love myself', results in a quick and ready treatment with drugs. Stress does produce psychological changes and drugs can give immediate relief but there is a danger that an overdosage of stimulants and antidepressants will lead to a build-up of anxiety or, vice versa, sedatives and hypnotics will reduce vigilance and efficiency while lessening the symptoms of anxiety. Drugs are obviously a popular solution for patient and doctor, judging from the vast quantities now prescribed, but they are generally only temporary solutions and fail to get at the cause; alternatively they may become habitual.

In psychiatry it is difficult in many cases to make a clear diagnosis. In physical medicine diagnoses are usually made, even when in doubt, but in psychological medicine there can be many varied causes for the onset of an illness. The whole personality and experience has to be taken into account and psychopathological tests are unreliable. Often too, the stressed person is acutely conscious of a social stigma being attached to changes in behaviour which cannot be attributed to some physical cause. Sometimes patients attending the day centre say they are 'going for physio' or 'regular check-up'. One patient after many weeks of daily attendance and ostensibly thirty years of a 'good' marriage still tells his wife he is attending the rehabilitation centre.

Given referral for treatment, problems can arise from the different theoretical bases from which therapists can operate, unless there is close interprofessional communication and a united multi-disciplinary team. There is a danger of conflict between them resulting in lack of consistency in working with the patient. Take for example the confusion which could exist in the treatment of a patient if the nurse encouraged his dependency and allowed regressed behaviour, if the psychologist was satisfied with the successful accomplishment of a very clearly defined task, if the psychiatrist was embarking on intensive psychotherapy and if the occupational therapist was pushing the patient to take responsibility and develop more mature forms of behaviour.

The above is somewhat exaggerated and it is probably more likely that, although aims of treatment for individual patients will differ within and between groups, some generalisations can be made. The patient learns that he is accepted. He develops positive self-regard and is given verbal approval as and when appropriate; it may be a warm welcoming hug from staff each day or a one-to-one discussion. Opportunities are created for him to test out reality, to look at his distorted ideas and learn to discriminate between the rational and irrational. What really does happen to the patient who fears that 'No one will ever speak to me again if I tell you what the real problem is'? Thus, through discussion and role playing, frightening ideas can be examined, attacked, and alternative forms of dealing with them practised. However, while learning new approaches it must be borne in mind that the patient's unconscious needs which initiated the original maladaptive behaviour cannot be ignored and must be satisfied in some other way. The patient must learn that he can be effective and in control, that negativism is destructive and that positive attitudes reinforce the agreeable responses of others towards him. He has to learn that depression and helplessness will not gain him sympathy. Indeed in the anti-depression room in Veterans Administration Hospital, Alabama (Taulbee & Wright, 1971) every action of the patient is criticised and condemned. If he sands the wood one way it is wrong: if he sands it the other way it is still wrong. Thus is he harrassed until he responds with anger: to which staff apologise and he is allowed out of the room. Having been forced into responding to his circumstances, he gains control and an alleviation of his helpless depression. Overt anger and depression cannot co-exist.

In a well-organised treatment centre there will be a consensus of opinion about approaches to treatment and the desirable goals for the patients, but consideration does also need to be given to the effectiveness of individual members of staff. Therapists, of whatever ilk, need to be members of a team with the ability to communicate with each other and to share ideologies. But because therapists are also human, each will bring his or her own specific skills and personal strengths and weaknesses. Mental health is just as important for staff as it is for patients, and is the result of successful interpersonal relationships where stress can be coped with independently or through the support of others or through the use of sensitivity and T-groups for staff.

However, not only trained staff are in a position to help those with psychological problems. Patients can also fulfil a therapeutic role by support, empathising or providing appropriate reinforcement when another achieves a desired goal. Indeed, Maxwell Jones (1968) claimed that patients themselves should decide how their fellow patients should be treated, and it is my experience that patients will often be the strongest confronters and shrewdest analysers of a distressed person's behaviour. In view of the fact that a number of patients return for treatment over a period of years, it is inevitable that they became exposed to, and pick up, therapeutic skills which they are able to use to the advantage of others. If only they could apply them to themselves—but then theory is easier, so often, than practice.

Conclusion

It is difficult to draw firm conclusions about the advantages and disadvantages of professional intervention. However, on a personal level I would hardly be writing this chapter if I did not believe in the therapeutic contribution of occupational therapists and others. When a patient has to be admitted to hospital, the quiet therapeutic environment can offer much to help him come to terms with his difficulties. At the same time, he is being removed from that very situation precipitating the stress. Change, as escape, can help restore the body's energies but this same change, if too long, can reduce confidence to face the real world. Thus, hospitalisation can become a reinforcer of the sick role of dependent behaviour unless the staff take active steps to avoid this. Yet the bureaucratic hierarchy of large mental hospitals often defeats the purpose for which it exists and, instead of encouraging flexibility, it expects patients to conform to a clearly defined social system where uniforms demarcate status and there is a power structure bearing little resemblance to life outside. However, a large institution does have many resources to draw upon, whereas the small nucleus of permanent staff is very vulnerable to the loss of even just one member. At the same time, it is easier for a small staff to communicate and share in treatment ideals. In a small flexible unit the patients too can help take responsibility for each other and so for themselves. After all, since it would appear that those most able to cope with stress are those who value themselves, have the ability to externalise unhappy feelings and are able to take responsibility for their actions, then this is what should be aimed at for those more vulnerable. There are no easy answers to this controversial subject, for our vulnerability is part of the essence of being human.

REFERENCES

Berne E 1964 Games people play. Grove Press, New York
Birtchnell J 1970 Early parental death & mental illness. British Journal of Psychiatry 116: 281–313
Bruhn J G 1962 Broken homes amongst attempted suicides and psychiatric outpatients. Journal of Mental Service 108: 772–779
Earle A M, Earle B V 1961 Early maternal deprivation and later psychiatric illness. American Journal of Orthopsychiatry 31: 181–186
Eysenck H J, Rachman S 1970 Dimensions of personality. In: Semenoff B (ed) Personality assessment
Hathaway S R, McKinley J C 1951 Excerpts from MMPI manual, Psychological Corporation. In Semenoff B (ed) 1970 Personality assessment. Penguin, Harmondsworth
Jones M 1968 Social psychiatry in practice. Penguin, Harmondsworth
Levitt E 1971 The psychology of anxiety. Paladin, London
Rutter M 1966 Children of sick parents: an environmental and psychiatric study. Oxford University Press, Oxford
Rutter M et al 1975 Helping troubled children. Penguin, Harmondswhorth
Seligman M 1975 Helplessness. W H Freeman, San Francisco
Spitz R A 1945 Hospitalism: an inquiry into the genesis of psychiatric conditions in early childhood. Psychoanalytic Studies of Children 1: 53–74
Taulbee E S, Wright H W 1971 A psychosocial-behavioural model for therapeutic intervention. In: Spielberger C D (ed) Current topics in clinical and community psychology III. Academic Press, New York
Thatcher D 1980 The slower learner. Unpublished work.
Walton H J 1958 Suicidal behaviour in depressive illness. Journal of Mental Science 104: 884–891

RECOMMENDED READING

Beck A T 1970 Cognitive therapy: nature and relation to behaviour therapy. Behaviour Therapy 1: 184–200

Beech H R (Ed) 1974 Obsessional states. Methuen & Co Ltd, London
Granville-Grossman K 1982 Recent advances in clinical psychiatry—4. Churchill Livingstone, Edinburgh
Munro A 1969 Parent–child separation. Archive of General Psychiatry 20: 598–604
Orford J 1976 The social psychology of mental disorder. Penguin, Harmondsworth
Sharpe R, Lewis D 1977 Thrive on stress. Souvenir Press, London

3

Diana Grellier

Physical dysfunction

INTRODUCTION

There is nothing new in the concept that patients with physical illnesses may have existing, associated or acquired psychological problems. The amount of time, emphasis and skill that is given to recognising or dealing with these problems is variable and dependent on the knowledge and interest of the therapist. Although we as occupational therapists are trained to look at the patient as a 'whole' and spend half of our training studying normal and abnormal psychology, many of us do not seem to be able to transfer our skills which relate to psychiatry to our treatment of physically ill people. Maybe this is related in part to historical attitudes in medicine and environmental factors within each institution and in part to the personality and preferences of the therapist who chooses a specific area of work. Perhaps too, some therapists choose a post where it is assumed there will be no emotional involvement.

This chapter is included to encourage another look at some of the problems arising from physical illness or handicap and, in conjunction with the rest of the text, may promote further consideration of how a therapist may use knowledge and skills learned in psychiatry with patients affected primarily by physical symptoms.

The psychiatric bias

It would seem that in psychiatry the main focus of the therapist's attention is directed towards the secondary handicaps exhibited by patients. In a physical setting the therapist's bias appears to be directed more towards the primary handicaps of the patient, which are the mechanical problems which arise from that illness or disease and which affect the patient's functional performance with everyday skills. To do full justice to a patient's treatment it should be remembered that it is just as important to consider or be clear about

53

dicaps which consist of non-adaptive reactions to ich differ between individuals who have the same lity. The attitudes of others can also affect, either ufavourably, the patient's own attitudes and behaviowards himself and others, his illness and treatment, his future, and his personal and social life. How he copes with illness, stress and change will be dependent on his premorbid personality. The therapist therefore needs to have equal awareness of these factors and be able to take them into account when setting goals for treatment.

To assist the patient to come to terms with his disability it may require, for instance, more conscious thought from the therapist to recognise and appreciate the patient's effort to succeed in a task, and its importance to the patient, or to recognise when positive re-enforcement is required if motivation is to be perpetuated. Conversely, the therapist should remember the importance of good assessment to ensure that the patient does succeed in tasks set. How important too is the environment in which the treatment is given? This can often play a more effective part than is given credence in a physical department.

Psychiatrically based activities

There appears to be a need to consider more broadly some of the techniques and activities associated with psychiatry and described within books such as this one. Most physical activities are concerned with the functional use of the limbs, with no cognizance of the psychological problems or primary needs of the individual. It would seem there is a place for creative therapies to encourage self-expression or the externalisation of problems not yet faced so that the patient can come to terms with himself or with a handicap. Perhaps counselling skills, too, need to be more readily available for patients and families from those who have most contact and who elicit the most trust. How many 'professionals' make it their business or have time to stop, listen, chat or explain? We talk about gaining 'rapport' with the patient but do we fully realise the significance and value of this statement? How much training or how many facilities are available to the physically handicapped for increasing social competence as part of the developmental process or in the adjustment of a new 'role' or 'image'? How, too, is anxiety managed? Thoughts on the type and use of activities, the priorities and needs of the patient and the attitudes and insight of the therapist to the psychological problems associated with physical illness are all areas of concern if the patient is to get maximum benefit from treatment.

TRAUMA

Physiological shock following a sudden physical trauma is well recognised and attended to by first-aid treatment available at 'ground-level' through to specialised units concerned, for example, with burns, spinal and coronary care. The psychological consequences of these and other conditions, from admission through to discharge, do not often afford the same attention for the patient from the 'professionals'.

This section is, therefore, concerned with the psychological features that may result from sudden physical trauma and loss, which may affect the patient at different stages of recovery and which may have a profound affect upon the outcome of his ability to cope with the consequences of and adaptation to disability.

By sudden physical trauma is meant some misfortune or unexpected happening which changes a person from being 'normal' one moment to a 'patient' the next. If it is easier, think of this as being yourself. One's interpretation of normality lies in the development of a self-concept which is derived from one's own and from others' perceptions. How we are viewed in different contexts and the nature of our relationships with family, friends and colleagues has a known significance. In *this* context we have plans for today and maybe long term plans for tomorrow. There is an order, familiarity and pattern in our existence which is taken for granted and which also brings a measure of security to our 'being'.

Accidents cause trauma. 'Internal' accidents, are the result of physiological disorder or disease and can result for example in coronary heart disease or cerebral vascular accidents. 'External' accidents can be the result of one's own or another's inattention, ignorance or lack of judgement. For instance, if a tree falls down in a gale and hurts someone it may be the result of ignorance, if the owner did not know that it was diseased, or bad luck in that someone was passing at that particular moment. Road traffic accidents, the cause of many and multiple injuries, are often the result of risk, inattention or bad judgement and involve one or more parties. Damage may include fractures, spinal, head and soft tissue injuries or crush injuries that require amputation. Sporting, domestic and work-related accidents also occur through one's own or another's folly with devastating results. All age groups are involved. The resulting damage may be interpreted by the 'affected' as unnecessary and futile as in war, or else as being one's own or another's fault. Whatever the cause the result is sudden and unexpected, altering instantly the pattern of one's life.

Effects on the patient

Pre-existing factors. Emotional stress has a known influence on physical health and contributes to physical illness. Hypertension, a predisposing cause of cardiovascular disease, is one example of a physical factor which is closely related to anxiety and emotional turmoil or the inhibition of angry feelings. Social stress and upheaval also put strain and pressure on the individual. In addition to these, Totman (1979) believes that each person has 'social rules' which he adheres to. Failure to do so following a life event or crisis puts the person at risk of physical illness. Inattention, a cause of 'external' accident, can be the result of many things, such as fatigue, over-indulgence of alcohol, anxiety related to work, home or personal matters but all are symptoms of stress. The earlier influence of stress on the patient and past life experiences, personality traits, family and cultural values which were a part of the patient prior to the accident, will all affect the individual's adjustment to trauma.

Following trauma. The psychological effects on the patient will be determined by the circumstances surrounding the accident, preexisting factors and the nature and severity of the injury. With brain damaged patients there is no reason to believe that they do not go through the same reactions as other patients following trauma, only that these reactions may be increased or decreased according to the involvement or severity of comprehension, interpretation or communication difficulties.

Hospitalisation/admission. It should be remembered that, on admission, everything for the patient is new and unfamiliar, including his own physical state. The atmosphere is clinical. The rules and rituals related to the treatment and hospital routine are unknown. The patient is stripped of identity by the removal of familiar clothes, and in the nakedness in which some have to be nursed there is further loss of dignity and self-esteem. He, the patient, is unknown to staff, and he does not know them. From bed the world may be viewed from the horizontal position, and this view may even be limited, fixed or rotated by others as in the nursing of spinal injuries. Privacy is invaded. All or many physical needs may have to be attended to by others. This is made worse if control of personal functions has also been lost. Decisions are taken by others, and the patient's opinion is no longer sought. The patient is isolated by distance from normal contact with others and the 'outside world' or by communication difficulties due to injury or life-saving devices. The patient can become defenceless in his need for help and as a result of the 'role' that he has now been given. Will he become irreversibly dependent in time too?

Emotional responses

Stages of adjustment to disability have been described as including shock, mourning, denial, acknowledgement and adaptation. Lindemann (1981) states that stages of reaction are more sharply defined in the case of traumatic injury due to the sudden nature of the damage. For instance following spinal cord injury the responses are shock, denial, anger, depression and acceptance or adjustment.

Shock. Lindemann also suggests that shock, as a protective mechanism, occurs over a relatively short period of time. It should be remembered however that during this period the family can feel as much or more overwhelming anxiety and fear than the patient. For the patient it may be a short period of psychological disorientation, but for the family a period of crisis.

Anxiety. It is common for anxiety to accompany physical illness. Initial concerns may be related to whether he, the patient, will recover or how the family will manage. As the patient becomes increasingly egocentric and somatically preoccupied, he may become afraid that he is going out of his mind or worry continuously about the possible outcome of his illness. On the other hand anxiety about some aspect of his illness may become out of proportion to the more realistic concerns of present and future. Some patients may find it unacceptable to externalise feelings and fears. Yet anxiety can interfere with the patient's co-operation in treatment, or reduce the energy that is needed for rehabilitation.

Bereavement. Following physical loss or damage it is a natural response to grieve, but it is also a necessary part of the process if a patient is to come to terms with the changes in self-concept and body image. It is sometimes forgotten that families mourn the sudden absence of their partner or the apparent loss of the personality previously known to them, for they too are affected by the physical change or loss.

Anger is a response to 'why should it have happened to me', the unfairness and the 'hurt' of being in this situation. If it includes 'look how it will affect my future', then this, in itself, is part of the process of recognising that change will have to take place. Often patients become angry about the attitudes of staff to their predicament, which may or may not be justified. Usually, there is a target for their anger such as the staff, the family, the employer or an organisation. Families too can feel anger and give vent to it. Expressive forms of this include verbal abuse, sudden rage or physical violence. If anger is not recognised by the patient and externalised then he may become sullen, hostile or depressed. Further internalisation may be self destructive.

Depression is associated with feelings of hopelessness and the inability to cope. This is further perpetuated by feelings of inadequacy and dependency. The depth of depression may be increased by guilt, especially if the accident involved others, or if irrational feelings of anger have been directed towards those upon whom the patient is dependent. The patient, an independent person, may now view himself permanently in a disabled role, or be aware of his lack of effectiveness in his previous role. Depression is usually associated with early stages on the 'road to recovery' and intermittently after this, and in varying forms of intensity. Only when it persists in unexpected cases and conditions may help be needed. Depression may be a recognised feature of some conditions. For example, it is frequently seen in cases of left-sided brain damage and in those stroke victims who fail to resume social activities. 'Home coming depression' is common in those who have suffered a myocardial infarction.

Denial. It may be 'nature's way' for there to be a gradual consciousness of the effects of disability and loss, so that as the patient becomes stronger 'inside and out' they can come to terms with a new self-concept and body image. Initially, denial is a protective defence mechanism, but when it persists maladaptive reactions may take the form of 'everything will be alright when I get home' or similar totally unrealistic comments. Sometimes patients can be too jovial, which may indicate that they have not yet begun to come to terms with their problems. The gradual process of total denial to acceptance may take a long time.

Maladaptive responses. Progress towards adjustment or adaptation to disability may be halted by various unconscious defences that protect individuals but which keep them in 'limbo'. Overt physical and emotional dependency, regression to childlike levels of maturity, repression of feelings so that they are not brought to consciousness and fantasising unrealistic solutions to problems, are all forms of defence. Other forms of defence may be excess of anxiety, unplaced anger which leads to negative behaviour and responses, depression which is perpetuated even to self-destruction, and denial of the situation to the extent of non-acceptance.

Adjustment and acceptance

Moos and Tsu (1977) describe seven major stages in the acquisition of coping skills which lead to adjustment and acceptance:

The first stage involves denying or minimising the seriousness of the illness, through the use of defence mechanisms.

The second stage includes seeking relevant information and learning about the disability.

The third stage is a request for reassurance and emotional support from family, friends and staff.

The fourth stage is learning about the specific illness-related procedures, as in the use of a wheelchair.

The fifth stage includes setting manageable goals which are evolved from smaller parts taken from overwhelming problems.

The sixth stage involves rehearsing alternative outcomes which prepare for difficulties that may be encountered, and which allay anxiety.

The seventh and final stage is a coping skill which arrives out of finding a general purpose, pattern and meaning to things and which enables a direction to be set as a perspective is found.

DETERIORATING DISEASES

Trauma is of sudden origin. This section is concerned with diseases of a deteriorating nature which may have no known cause and where there is little or no hope of a successful cure. Often there is uncertainty over the diagnosis, especially if there is no genetic cause or there has been a delay in diagnosis because earlier symptoms were not associated with the disease or thought relevant, or because the cause of them has been rationalised by the person concerned and an opinion was not sought. Sometimes reported symptoms have led a person to be labelled neurotic or even psychotic before the true nature of their disease has been exposed.

With neurological diseases, such as multiple sclerosis, muscular dystrophy or motor neurone disease, patients may have had indications of sensory change or clumsiness over a period of time, or intermittently, before the symptoms have been recognised. In rheumatoid arthritis the patient may, for instance, have had problems with sight, before the more tell-tale signs of general malaise and joint involvement were apparent. With malignancies the condition may have suddenly come to light through the presence of a blockage or palpable lump, as opposed to the more insidious beginnings of leukaemia or Hodgkin's disease. Prior to diagnosis the patient may have gone through uncertain and unhappy patches and may only in hindsight have realised that they had not been feeling well for some time, but that they had not been aware of the fact. For those where a hereditary illness is known to exist within the family, fear, denial or anticipation may have been there long before the early symptoms were exhibited—as in Huntington's Chorea.

Only when the disease is diagnosed will the patient or family be told. The course of the disease may be unpredictable and it may not be known how it will specifically affect that patient. The frequency of visits to the hospital, or time span between home and hospital, will also be unknown, as will the speed with which the symptoms may advance. It should also be remembered that these diseases affect the entire body and life style of the patient, and may affect the personality as in Huntington's chorea or mood as in Parkinson's disease.

Risk factors in the cause of illness

As has been said earlier in the chapter, the way in which people react to stress, both emotionally and psychologically, affects their susceptibility to physical illness. Totman (1979) discusses the ideas of others on the loss–disease hypothesis, and the incidence of illness following this type of experience. Loss is not necessarily felt only as the result of a death or separation, but also after such experiences as the menopause, a rejection by someone upon whom one was dependent, desertion, eviction, the arrival of a rival sibling, or the threat of separation. It has been noted that these losses can give rise to feelings of hopelessness or despair, as in the case of patients who develop leukaemia. Contrary to this, it could be argued that due to the frequency of life stresses, the chance of finding an incidence of stress prior to illness is high and therefore not significant.

Hereditary factors are considered to be relevant and are a contributory factor in some diseases such as cancer, although research in this field is inconclusive. The correlation of certain types of personality and susceptibility to certain diseases has been much written about but is still unsupported, there being insufficient evidence. Richards (1982) for instance, admits that he supports the axiom that happy, outgoing people are less likely to get cancer, than their introverted opposites. From his experience he has found that many patients diagnosed were restrained by habit, were shy, nervous, discontented, low sexed and had a congenital lack of drive and initiative. Elizabeth Forsyth (1979) a GP who contracted multiple sclerosis says of herself and other sufferers that they are energetic and hardworking people, with a tendency to overwork and to having bouts of energy. Jean Atkinson (1974), another sufferer, notes with humour that many patients with multiple sclerosis were born in January, but I am sure the scientists will never be convinced by the linking of sunsigns with health.

Totman suggests that another contributory factor to be considered may be 'social incongruity'. For instance, it has been noted that there is a high incidence of this in parents of women with rheumatoid arthritis. Social incongruity is defined as a different social status between married partners, which puts stress on the partner who has to function out of his or her normal social circle.

Geographical areas are also associated with high incidence of certain diseases and it is unknown whether this is due to racial, dietary, or atmospheric factors. E. Forsyth makes the point that the more passive Roman Catholics of southern Europe who live in a milder climate and who are oil eaters and wine drinkers are less tense, driving and compulsive characters than their northern neighbours, who eat animal fat, drink beer, are probably Protestants and are more prone to multiple sclerosis. Is it the same analogy which makes the Swiss particularly prone to the disease?

It would appear that stress and emotion that is internalised makes some people more susceptible to physical illness than others. How a person reacts to his illness will affect its length and course. Those with positive attitudes, and who have a strong will against the disease often live longer and more happily, in spite of all the difficulties which are in their way.

Effect on the patient and family

Stages of reaction leading to acceptance and adjustment were described earlier in relation to trauma. Those reactions apply equally well to those who have a deteriorating or intractable disease diagnosed, although they may be less well defined and the process more gradual. Therefore, that information should be read in context with and seen to be contributory to this section. In both cases, the general pattern of reaction is subject to much variation, depending on the nature and course of the disability, the age and personality of the patient, the family and other medical, individual and social factors. Those reactions which are mostly considered normal and should be recognised for what they are, have also been referred to as phases of bereavement. The coming to terms with the loss of what one was, with what one is now and what one feels, leads to changes in body image, self-esteem and role. It may also be interesting to note that Lindeman (1981) observed that families of chronically ill people developed a perspective over a period of time, which made their reactions to the disability less intense than in cases of those with traumatic injuries.

Receiving the diagnosis

To receive such a diagnosis as described above must be a devastating experience at any stage of the illness. For a child born handicapped, the news has to be accepted by the parents. Initially, the reaction may be of overwhelming shock, bewilderment or disbelief or a combination of some or all of them. The significance of the news may be too much for the parents to take in or realise, or it may be hoped that 'it' may just go away. The immediate reaction may be to seek a second opinion to prove that the doctor was wrong or that the signs and symptoms indicate a more acceptable diagnosis. Further opinions may be sought especially when uncertainty over the diagnosis has been indicated or there is refusal to accept the inevitable. Only once the diagnosis has been accepted can more positive steps be taken towards adjustment.

For some families there may be the added dilemma of when to tell the truth to the person affected. For the patient who already knows, his dilemma may be of when to tell those 'near' him. How to do it creates another factor. Perhaps, we should stop sometimes and wonder how we would cope in these circumstances? For one partner to know and the other not to may put additional strain on the relationship.

Reacting to knowledge

Once the significance becomes apparent further knowledge may be sought, for example from libraries or general practitioners or 'the lady down the road' who 'knows you know'. This may be in the hope of finding comfort to contradict what one was beginning to believe, or for a greater knowledge of the truth to be faced.

Many patients can feel tearful, emotional and easily upset in the early days after a diagnosis has been given. Relationships, too may become strained, especially in the initial stages, or later, if 'coming to terms with things' is uneven, when one partner denies the truth while the other one realises the consequences and may even over-react.

For those who are not passive in their acceptance of knowledge there are feelings of bitterness and anger, especially if they can consciously allow themselves to feel this emotion. For many this is the start of a fight against their illness which continues to the very end, while for others fate is accepted readily, apathetically or negatively.

Changes in mood may be as much due to coming to terms with the condition when realisation sets in, as the restrictions and frustrations that the illness increasingly imposes, whether this be tiredness, fatigue, slowness, uncoordination, stiffness, tremor, difficulties with initiation of movement, poor sight, incoherent speech, sensory loss, dependence or the loss of the ability to carry out or continue previous skills. Some patients feel increasingly depressed to the point of feeling suicidal. There is a strong link between pain and depression or depression associated with specific illnesses or circumstances. The link between euphoria and multiple sclerosis may be more related to a non-acceptance syndrome of the disease process, hence the levels of depression felt by other sufferers who have accepted the situation. Changes in personality traits may be one of the hardest things to face or to fear, especially if this is known to be associated with the disease.

From fear to anxiety, there must be many questions that come to mind for the patient.

Will I be able to do next year what I can do now?
Will my essential relationships survive the next downward move?
How can I cope with depression?
Will I live or die—or how can I face death?
Will my personality survive?
How can I retain control over my behaviour and future?
Can I cope with decreasing independence?
Can I cope with pain?

For the family the questions may be:

Can I cope with the thought that they will be different?
Am I independent enough to cope—or able?

Do I want to be able to cope?
Who is there who will help me?
What will it mean to our relationship?
How will the family manage?

Consequences

Following the physical crisis of trauma there is an element of hope of improvement or of intervention to make permanent improvements. For the patient with a deteriorating disease there is not that hope, only a downward pattern to be adapted to as changes take place. There may be speedy down trends during exacerbations or flare-ups before a levelling out or plateau when suddenly everything seems alright, possibly for ever. The pattern of life is lost from time to time if hospitalisation is required and the patient loses the much needed security of the home.

As the patient has to cope with increasing dependence, so the family has to cope with increasing independence or dependence on outside help.

DISFIGUREMENT

There are many things which add up to disfigurement and to which we react, but which those affected have to accept and make the best of. These may vary from a pimple on the end of the nose, to a squint, to severe scarring following burns or soft tissue injury, to congenital or acquired deformity, to stages before, between or after plastic or reconstructive surgery, to the amputation of a part or whole of a limb, or to multiple handicap. Often in the long term it may be more difficult for the person affected to cope with others and their reactions, than with coming to terms with the physical abnormality.

Appearance

Thousands and millions of pounds are spent annually by individuals on the enhancement of their appearance whether it be on clothes, make-up, hair fashion, or the removal or disguise of blemishes. The importance of appearance stems from the fact that we wish to be sexually and socially attractive and very definitely acceptable to others in many ways. We also wish to convey impressions of how we think we are, or would like to be seen. For example, the person who wishes to appear virile and totally healthy may avoid wearing glasses by spending ill-afforded money on contact lenses. Beauty is therefore something to be admired and aimed for, as beauty indicates perfection and completeness, and promises satisfaction with oneself and from others. Those disfigured start disadvantaged, and money cannot buy the perfection sought by others. Bodily imperfections also lead to dissatisfaction in oneself.

The attitudes of others

People's attitudes to the disfigurement and unattractive appearance of others are automatic, quite unconscious, and lead to a stigma for the disabled as evidence that this person is emotionally unstable and intellectually limited. They do not in fact 'match up' to those that are not blemished, so that a visible handicap is seen to represent incompleteness inside as well as out. Our immediate reaction to meeting disability and disfigurement is often negative, there being initially a feeling of horror and disgust, which might then be followed by the recognition that sympathy should really have been felt. For the 'affected' they have to cope with these reactions and accept them. It is also known that we fear that we ourselves may be or become different. We are affected by the prejudices and the interpretations we give to those differences in others. We see ourselves as others see us, so for the disfigured their self-concept is affected by our attitudes and reactions.

For those disfigured

Disability for a disfigured person is in communication and social interaction. The more visible a handicap the more socially destructive. The disability may become the focus of attention for either party, or else denied or conspicuously avoided. Interaction may be limited to a few social 'niceties' and the person affected will have to explore or expect that they may either be rejected because of 'stigma' or accepted through enlightenment.

Those facially disfigured are further disadvantaged in social interactions involving communication. Visual problems may exclude proper eye to eye contact. To make contact the eyes and the face become the focus of attention so that any blemish, however small, is brought instantly to another's awareness. Bad disfigurements hide expression of what is being communicated and also of what a person may be like 'underneath'. Their face cannot be hidden only noticed. To deny this type of disfigurement may lead a person to flaunt their 'scars' without undue awareness of the effect on others. To be over conscious of the effects on others, leads to social withdrawal or families hiding the 'affected' offspring. To survive or to establish or maintain a variety of 'roles' however changed, means interaction with others whether at home, at the shops, at work or at play. Because of the stigma surrounding appearance, and therefore the reaction of 'others' which includes the public, job opportunities are also restricted.

This also applies to those with hand disfigurements, which affect the unacknowledge part of the personality, for we shake hands with others in greeting to express thanks, or touch others to show affection. Abnormal hands may also affect a means of expression. Hands are also always before us and others. It may therefore be more comfortable to 'pocket' them away. How often there must be conflict for surgeons and their patients in deciding whether, for instance, to make or reconstruct a hand to become more functional at the expense of cosmetic loss, so the patient can become more independent, or be able to work, to satisfy that 'role'. Is it worse to be born with a disfigurement or to acquire it, or are both equally psychologically disabling for different reasons, including those related to age?

Stature

There must be some significance in the interpretation of height in oneself or others. People who are small seem to make up for it in other ways. Is it that we become more aware of their personality and drive because of their absence of height or is it that they feel they have to compensate for their lack of stature because we expect more from those 'higher'? Women who are particularly tall, on the other hand, often stoop or wear shoes with flat heels, while some men who are short appear to welcome fashions in shoes that allow platform soles to be worn.

What therefore is the effect due to congenital abnormalities, illness or surgery where there is a loss in height, this being particularly relevant to those who are confined to a wheelchair? Many of the points raised under the heading of 'appearance' also apply to those with limited stature, or who are wheelchair-bound. For instance, how often is the attendant with a wheelchair user spoken to by a stranger to interpret and receive comments, as the occupier of the wheelchair is assumed to be unable to talk or communicate in acceptable terms? Maybe too, it is assumed that the personality and social abilities of the affected person are diminished.

What seems rarely understood is that the wheelchair owner has to learn skills to enable co-operation from the public and others if they are to become independent and normal. For instance, it may be possible to drive a car, but the ability to get a chair out of a car and position it appropriately may need the assistance of a 'passer by'. To communicate the help required, without arousing undue sympathy or over- or under-reaction, within acceptable bounds, needs self-confidence and ability. Too much help will be embarrassing, but it may fulfil the need of the 'other' as disability indicates dependency and helplessness. A negative reaction will also be unacceptable.

To be superior in height over another gives some people a feeling of power, of being able to 'look down upon' the other person, hence the reason why some people, in some situations, contrive to ensure that they are higher. This can give an appearance of, or feeling of, superiority. To reverse the situation, to be lower or reduced in stature than another may make for feelings of insignificance or insecurity, especially if 'others' use their height to stoop to communicate or to make the 'lower' feel inferior.

Movement

It has been found that those with functional impairment, who have conditions which are not responsive to medical intervention and which are of a permanent nature, rank lower in public acceptability than those people with an organic impairment, ulcer sufferers being the highest ranked and cerebral palsy sufferers the lowest. Siller et al (1967) ranked eight conditions in this order: deafness, blindness, amputation, skin disorders, paralysis, body deformations, muscular dystrophy and cerebral palsy. Jonathan Miller (1978) says that for the patient paralysis is an observable sign which represents for him a failure of what he regards should be his normal repertoire of power. Loss of or gradual restriction in movement means a reduction of independence and a need for dependence on others. Gillis (1980) says that some will fight against this to a point of over-independency, especially if deep down they know they could relapse into utter dependence, while others may regress quickly to a childlike state of dependency.

To become slower makes one out of 'tempo' with the rest of the world which is moving faster. People often do not have time to wait. Not only may it frustrate the 'affected' but also those on whom demands are being made. For the former athelete or physical fitness fanatic it is even worse. As with other handicaps individuals with similar problems often 'club' together to be with their 'own', these being others with similar or common problems. The reverse too may happen, when the last thing a person requires is to be linked or associated with those who are in a comparable situation. To feel comfortable and accepted it may therefore be necessary to be with one's 'own' or with the 'wise', the carers who have understanding and empathy (Willson, 1983).

Solutions

Only time, input and contact will improve the public image of the disabled and their automatic response. Meanwhile the disfigured need help. Burns (1980) argues that the professionals with a positive self-concept have more to offer than others. Are these characteristics looked for by those selecting potential students for the caring professions, and does the training encourage this completeness in students? Primarily those affected need positive input to alter their self-concept and self-esteem and to have the opportunity to come to terms with their limitations. They have to negotiate the boundaries of their disability or illness within the context of the stigma applied by society and the 'not knowing' of some of the professionals.

REFERENCES

Atkinson J 1974 Multiple sclerosis: a concise summary for nurses and patients. John Wright and Sons, Bristol
Burns R B 1980 Essential psychology. MTP Press, Lancaster
Forsyth E 1979 Living with multiple sclerosis. Faber and Faber, London
Gillis L 1980 Human behaviour in illness. Faber and Faber, London
Lindemann J E 1981 Psychological and behavioural aspects of physical disability. Plenum Press, New York
Miller J 1978 The body in question. Jonathan Cape, London
Moos R H, Tsu V D 1977 The crisis of physical illness: an overview. In: Moos R M (ed) Coping with physical illness. Plenum Press, New York
Richards D 1982 The topic of cancer. Pergamon Press, Oxford
Siller J et al 1967 Studies in reactions to disability XI: attitudes towards the physically disabled. New York University, New York
Totman R 1979 Social causes of illness. Souvenir Press Ltd, London
Willson M 1983 Occupational therapy in long term psychiatry. Churchill Livingstone, Edinburgh

RECOMMENDED READING

Atkinson R L, Atkinson R C, Hilgard E R 1983 Introduction to psychology.
Harcourt Brace Jovanovick, New York
Bernstein N R 1976 Emotional care of the facially burned and disfigured. Little,
Brown and Co., Boston
Curran D, Partridge M, Storey P 1980 Psychological medicine, 9th edn. Churchill
Livingstone, Edinburgh
Degre-Coustry C, Grevisse M 1982 Psychological problems in rehabilitation after
myocardial infarction; non institutional approach. Advanced Cardiology 29:
126–131
Feibel J H, Springer C J 1982 Depression and failure to resume social activities
after stroke. Archives of Physical Medical Rehabilitation 63: 276–278
Ingamells K 1981 The hand. In: Turner A (ed) The practice of occupational
therapy. Churchill Livingstone, Edinburgh
Lavers A 1981 Remedial involvement in the management of patients with
Huntingdon's chorea. The Association to Combat Huntingdon's Chorea,
Hinckley, Leicestershire
McDaniel J W 1976 Physical disability and human behaviour. Pergamon Press,
Oxford
O' Sullivan S B, Cullen K E, Schmitz T J 1981 Physical rehabilitation evaluation
and treatment procedures. F A Davis, Philadelphia
Robinson R G, Price T R 1982 Post stroke depressive disorders; a follow-up
study of 103 patients. Stroke 13: 5: 635–41
Versluys H P 1983 Psychosocial adjustment to physical disability. In: Trombly
C A (ed) Occupational therapy for physical dysfunction. Williams and Wilkins,
Baltimore

Influences on therapy

PART II

Influences on therapy

Humanistic psychology

INTRODUCTION

Humanistic psychology as an approach to the study of people includes a number of different theories which are bound together by a particular view of 'the person'. This view focusses upon the development of human potentialities and accepts that the subjective experience of the individual is important. It is a comparatively recent school of thought in psychology founded mainly by Abraham Maslow (1908–1970), with other writers such as Rollo May and Carl Rogers making valuable contributions from their own experience and insights, thus furthering understanding. In contrast to the theories expounded elsewhere humanistic psychology is neither objectivistic, regarding the person as a machine, nor deterministic, believing the individual to be in the hapless grip of unconscious forces; instead it sees the person as a growing developing creating being, with the ability to take full self-responsibility. It is an optimistic view, for human nature is assumed to be essentially good and the individual is motivated by an innate force toward the goal of 'actualisation', that is, developing to the full the potential with which he or she is born. Psychological health is marked by the greater expansion of this drive which in turn creates or enhances the person. Because the individual always responds as a whole being, it is not possible to study small elements of isolated behaviour. One can only study the total person, for the whole is greater than the sum of the parts. John Rowan (1976) writes, 'It is a whole new way of looking at psychological science. It is a way of doing science which includes love, involvment and spontaneity, instead of systematically excluding them'. In this chapter we shall look at some of the roots of humanistic psychology, and then at the work of two men who have had a great impact upon present thinking. These are Abraham Maslow and Carl Rogers.

ORIGINS OF HUMANISTIC PSYCHOLOGY

Current theories usually have their roots in the past and may also be influenced by other ideas around at the time. Traces of phenomenology, some forms of existentialism and Self Theory can be found within the humanistic perspective. These ideas have percolated the Group Movement and are evident in certain types of small group work.

Phenomenology

Phenomenology is the theory of 'Phenomena', literally translated, 'appearances'. It is the method of enquiry adopted by the German philosopher Edmund Husserl (1859–1938) which postulates the importance of the object as perceived by the senses of the person i.e. what the object appears to be rather than what it really is, is what really counts. In other words, the subjective reality for an individual is of greater value than the objective reality, however distorted or erroneous. Phenomenological psychology starts with attention to the person's perceptions and experiences; how he represents, organises and interprets consciously the stimuli of external and internal events which he registers. To give a very simple example: I thought a car was going to hit me, that was my perception and I took evasive action as quickly as possible; my action was based upon my interpretation of events. Subsequently, I discovered I was wrong, I misperceived the incident, and by-passers had been puzzled by my peculiar behaviour which, to them, appeared wholly inappropriate, even bizzare, for their perception was different.

From my point of view my actions were rational, they were grounded in my perception of events, only afterwards did I realise my mistake and was left feeling rather foolish. Phenomenology emphasises the uniqueness of each person's experience and frame of reference, making it impossible to have a generalised view of human beings. Rogers (1959) writes 'There is one attitude which I hold, which I believe has relevance for the proper evaluation of any theory I might present. It is my belief in the fundamental predominance of the subjective. Man lives essentially in his own personal and subjective world, and even his most objective functioning, in science, mathematics, and the like, is the result of subjective purpose and subjective choice'.

The influence of existentialism

It is impossible to explain all the complexities of this body of thought as it is amorphous; shifting in emphasis as it has developed in different places in conjunction with other disciplines. Heidegger (1889–1976), a pupil of Husserl (1859–1938), is regarded as a founding father of existentialism in his attempt to find human beings a place in the world. Existentialists believe that human beings cannot escape freedom and that freedom goes hand in hand with responsibility. Unlike animals, people are capable of self-awareness, a unique capacity which allows them to transcend a present event or situation and enables them to think and choose with certain freedom. Increased awareness leads to greater freedom as possibilities are considered and choices made which involve the individual in creating their own existence and destiny. As May states (1953) 'Man is the being who can be conscious of, and therefore responsible for, his existence'. The freedom that each person has to make choices from a number of possibilities and not be certain of the outcome of decisions gives rise to anxiety, an essential part of living. Anxiety also arises from the uncertainty of the future and knowledge of death which emphasise the limitations of life. There is only a short time in which to completely become what one is able to become, an 'Authentic Being'. Existentialists believe that people are constantly searching for meaning and purpose in life and each person has to discover this for themselves. Failure to create meaningful relationships may result in loneliness, isolation, hopelessness and despair.

Ronald Laing (b. 1927) a British psychiatrist, no longer accepts traditional psychiatry, having been influenced strongly by existentialism.

The central idea of Laing's approach is that suffering is the result of not being true to oneself. Throughout life, particularly in response to others, we pretend , and in order to protect ourselves we pretend that we are not pretending, defending ourselves with the unconscious defence mechanisms of distortion, projection and denial. The individual becomes 'alienated' that is disassociated from personal experience. This pretending that one is someone other than the real self can give rise to splitting, and a number of false selves emerge. For Laing the purpose of therapy is to allow the person to recover a sense of identity and personal authenticity. One then becomes 'ontologically secure' and has a much greater sense of one's own identity which provides a sound base for encountering others and coping with life events.

The influence of 'groups'.

Since the Second World War there has been an explosion of special 'groups' of all kinds. They go by many names; 'T' groups (T standing for training) 'encounter' groups, sensory awareness groups. They all have different emphases and forms but have common conceptual underpinnings which are due in large part to the thinking of Kurt Lewin (1890–1947), Carl Rogers and Gestalt Psychology. Lewin, a Polish psychologist, who had emigrated to the United States, had established (with colleagues) groups in the Massachusetts Institute of Technology, in order to study how democratic attitudes could be developed in group members. Their studies demonstrated that democratic leadership was an effective style of leadership in Western society, reducing autocracy, rigidity and hierarchical strata.

One particular incident changed the whole course of the study of groups. In 1946, observers of the current course wished to discuss the progress of that day with the trainers. The trainee group members asked if they too could attend. At that time this was an unheard of action, and must have given rise to a good deal of anxiety, particularly to the trainers, but permission was granted. The result was a whole new dimension of group interaction between all the three sections of the course, participants, observers and trainers. It was a highly charged encounter, at times almost explosive, and went on well into the night. On the other hand it was exciting, valuable and a great learning experience for all involved. Honest feedback had occurred for the first time and this was considered so important that the participants requested further participation in their own programme. This approach became an integral part of what is now known as 'T' groups, and the first course organised on these lines took place in 1947, just after Lewin's death.

About the same time at the University of Chicago, Carl Rogers was experimenting in the use of groups for training counsellors. He felt that cognitive training was not what was required as most trainees were very well qualified academically. A different approach was thought to be more appropriate, so the leaders experimented with an intensive group experience where the participants met for several hours each day in order to better understand themselves, to study their attitudes, emotional reactions and how they related to each other. It was hoped that adopting this method would enable the participants to learn to be more effective in their relationships and subsequently to be more skilful as counsellors. The sharing together which occurred in this course proved to be a very powerful experience with therapeutic value. Ideas from both Lewin's work and that of Rogers have mingled over the years and can now be discerned in many types of groups within the human potential movement. They exist to promote the growth of awareness of each individual group member, of others and of interactional skills. Experience is shared and reflected upon together, facilitating greater confidence, spontaneity and freedom to be oneself.

This is a third root from which current humanistic psychology has evolved into a force which has wide application in many fields: firstly, in all kinds of education, from young people to professional groups such as clergy, counsellors and occupational therapists; secondly, in organisational psychology, theory and practice; and thirdly, psychotherapy in its many guises. Expressive activities are frequently used in conjunction with psychotherapy today, a method first used at the Esalen Institute in 1961, and one that is familiar to many occupational therapists.

THE CONTRIBUTION OF ABRAHAM MASLOW

Abraham Maslow was born in 1908 and spent his working life in the pursuit of increasing his understanding of 'psychological health'. In this way, he hoped not only to be able to add to the improvement of a person's life, but also contribute to the good of society. The whole healthy person was the subject of his studies, not discrete parts of behaviour, not psychodynamics, not the disturbed or maladjusted, but people who appeared to him to function well and cope with life. One of his quests was to discover what motivates people throughout life, on what basis do they choose their options. Maslow's position developed slowly over many years and was influenced by ideas of other psychologists in the field, such as Kurt Goldstein to whom he dedicated his book *'Toward a Psychology of Being* (Maslow, 1968). From his studies of both normal and exceptional people , those he considered to be 'fully functioning', Maslow noted that they displayed particular, common characteristics. These included a superior perception of reality and greater acceptance of themselves, of others and nature. Continuing studies led him to postulate a new philosophy of the person and a more hopeful, encouraging way of conceiving all aspects of human knowledge and behaviour based upon a belief in the innate nature which is not intrinsically evil but, in essence, neutral or good. 'Anger is in itself not evil, nor is fear, laziness or even ignorance. Of course these can and do lead to evil behaviour but they needn't.'

Maslow conceived a system of needs and their fulfilment as the motivation of human behaviour. From these needs a driving force emerges and it is the urge to satisfy these physical and psychological needs which directs behaviour, which in turn contributes to the growth of inherent potentials within the person. This inner force pushes the individual towards 'self-actualisation', that is the process of becoming fully oneself.

Deficiency and growth motivation

Maslow observed that any human action may spring from a number of motives which have varying degrees of consciousness. He classified these motives into two large groups. Those associated with maintaining the survival of the individual, he described as 'Deficiency motives' and those associated with the enhancement of life in the direction of self-actualisation he called 'growth motives'.

Deficiency motives

These motives operate upon the principle that if a person has discomfort, such as hunger, thirst, sex, insecurity or fatigue, action is initiated to alleviate the discomfort: for example, the hungry person searches for food, in this country that is fairly simple, most of us can go to the pantry; in an underdeveloped country that may be a major undertaking. The successful search for food satisfies a basic need which will then no longer dominate thought or action, until hours later when the body is once again low in sustenance. The tension which arose from the deficiency is reduced by eating. A tension reduction model of motivation is quite well understood and accepted in modern thought but it does not adequately explain all behavioural motives. The survival tendency maintains life; it does not in any way enhance it, but it is very powerful and can be regarded as part of the core of personality.

Growth motives

People are frequently moved to action which has little to do with satisfying basic needs such as hunger and thirst, but which appear to enable them to develop beyond their present condition. Sebastian Coe as an athlete is indulging in activities which stretch him, demand energy, effort and at times, considerable stress. His behaviour cannot be explained in terms of reducing tension, indeed he deliberately seeks it. Motivation, here, has much more to do with development and growth. Seb Coe has so developed his potential, physically, that he is one of the best athletes in the world. This is what Maslow believes growth motives give rise to. In healthy people, actions are motivated by the need to actualise the potential with which one is born, one's talents and capacities, and at the same time accept one's own unique intrinsic nature.

Hierarchy of needs

Maslow studied healthy people as they went about their daily business. He observed people at work, solving problems, buying insurance, running competitively, buying a car and other such common activities. He also spent time studying biographies of great people such as Lincoln and Schweitzer. He noted that patterns emerged in behaviour, at times one type of need predominated and gave rise to actions, and at other times different needs dominated behaviour. His observations lead to the proposal that motives could be catagorised in a hierarchical way, and only if the needs of the lower catagory were satisfied would the needs of higher levels emerge and determine behaviour. He considered the physiological needs to be lower, and these had to be met first before a person would be concerned about higher needs, and these emerged in a set order.

Physiological needs

These needs are concerned with maintaining the body physically. They include the need for warmth, oxygen, food, water and sex. If these needs are not met adequately, death will ensue, so behaviour is organised around those activities which will ensure their satisfaction. As these needs are met to an acceptable level, the next group of needs appears.

Safety needs

Safety needs are concerned with being secure from physical danger, the avoidance of pain and the maintainance of psychological security. A man threatened with redundancy is in no physical danger but is psychologically endangered as his future is extremely uncertain. Much of his behaviour will be motivated by the anxiety that arises from his position and will be directed to the alleviation of that anxiety. He will try to hang on to his present position, join union attempts to combat redundancies at the same time as looking for another job. The safety needs are preponderant and direct behaviour. Similarly, a child who lives in an environment with no consistent rules and boundaries will be unable to satisfy these needs and actions may be directed to finding greater security.

Belongingness and love needs

These are concerned with the satisfaction of needs of intimacy, the receiving and acceptance of trust, affection and pleasure one with another. Such needs emerge if the physiological and safety needs are reasonably gratified. A person in this state is very aware of the absence of friends and family and will strive to meet this need through activity directed to this goal. Neighbourhood friends, colleagues at work, friendships through leisure activities are all ways of satisfying these needs. The rapid increase of personal growth groups and 'T' groups in the last few decades may in part be due to an unsatisfied drive for intimate relationships which are no longer met in our mobile society where traditional groups are scattered or broken. Sex may be an element of these love needs as it is usually associated with the giving and receiving of love, but it can, as already indicated, be studied as a purely physiological need.

The esteem needs

Maslow recognised from his studies the need that people have to feel good about themselves. A person needs to have self-esteem and self-regard as well as esteem and regard for others. There is a desire for achievment, for meeting the challenge of mastering the environment, for competence and confidence to cope with the world. All these Maslow describes as esteem needs. From other people the individual needs recognition, regard, prestige, affirmation and appreciation which contribute to a growth of confidence, strength, coping abilities and feelings of self-worth. The thwarting of these needs leads to feelings of inferiority and helplessness. When all the needs associated with survival are satisfied, those associated with actualisation become salient.

The need for self-actualisation

As already mentioned, the goal of healthy living is self-actualisation, the process whereby one develops fully what one is potentially able to become. This way one can find peace with oneself, being true to one's own nature. Very few people are self actualisers according to Maslow, mainly because most people never satisfy the lower needs, although every person has the capacity for self-actualisation. These five groups are the basis of most action in people. Maslow did, however, discuss cognitive impulses and the need to explore the unknown in order to understand.

The desires to know and understand

Maslow (1954) was aware that human beings are often directed by a need to know, to find out, and satisfactory results from these searches leads to 'a bright emotional spot in a person's life'. Frustration, on the other hand, leads to boredom, loss of zest for life, self-dislike and general depression.

The aesthetic needs

Another group of needs that Maslow considered important were those to do with the appreciation of beauty, shape and form. There is evidence for this in all cultures, particularly amongst healthy children.
These last two groups do not fit neatly into the system of needs, but they are clearly closely linked.

Characteristics of self-actualising people

Maslow observed that there were common features in all people who were actualisers. He noted that all of them have:

1. Superior perception of reality which is not distorted by personal wants and needs.
2. A realistic acceptance of themselves, their strengths and weaknesses and of others and the natural world.
3. A greater spontaneity of expression.
4. A problem-solving approach to life rather than self-preoccupation.
5. A need for privacy and their higher autonomy means less dependence on others.
6. A vivid appreciation of things around them.

7. A spirituality, though not necessarily in the formal religious sense. They may also have 'Peak experiences' when they feel ecstatically powerful, transcendent and yet completely at one with the world.
8. Intimacy with a few well chosen friends of a deep nature.
9. Democratic values, open and spontaneous with others whoever they are.
10. A recognition of the difference between ends and means.
11. A sense of humour which is not hostile, more philisophical.
12. A capacity for creativity, original and fresh.
13. A certain nonconformity, resisting the cultural pressures.

This list is rather overwhelming so it is not surprising that Maslow considered very few people ever achieved such maturity. As you will see, this is very similar to Rogers' description of the 'fully functioning' person to be discussed later. Although there are many critics of Maslow's theory it has had a wide impact on current thinking and one that helps occupational therapists to understand the needs of patients or clients. We cannot expect the elderly person living alone to be very keen to return to the community where she knows from experience she manages with great difficulty to get out, follow a daily routine and rarely meets anyone. All these needs are more likely to be much more satisfactorily met in hospital. In hospital she can give attention to 'higher things', at home she is struggling to survive.

THE CONTRIBUTION OF CARL ROGERS

Carl Rogers' (b. 1902) approach to understanding arises not from the study of healthy people like Maslow's, but from his work as a therapist. He was born into a fairly strict religious family in Chicago, a fact which he described later in life as 'rather burdensome'. In his early years he was interested in the biological sciences, an interest which is evident in his later thinking. He left college (school) to enter the Union Theological Seminary of New York City, but did not stay long, moving to Columbia University to read Psychology where he was strongly influenced by the philosophy of John Dewey (1859–1952). His subsequent clinical studies, teaching and researches created in him a growing interest in personality and psychotherapy. In his initial clinical work he was exposed to Freudian thought but found himself much more in sympathy with theorists who emphasised the importance of one's view of one's 'self' as determining behaviour. Rogers' writings in the humanistic tradition are regarded as being the most articulate, comprehensive and systematic, and carry weight far beyond the boundaries of psychology. He presented his first formulation of his theory as an approach to therapy in *Client Centred Therapy* (1951) and later, in *On Becoming a Person* (1961). It is more formally presented in a chapter in Koch's *Psychology: A Study of a Science*.

Theoretical rationale

The self

Central to Rogers' theory is his concept of 'self'. The self is an organised set or pattern of perceptions, feelings, attitudes and values characteristic of the 'I' and the 'Me' which the individual being believes are uniquely his own. The term also includes perceptions held about others. It refers to the person's conscious sense of who and what he is, not what others experience him to be. The person's own subjective thoughts and feelings about himself are what is real for him, and it is these which direct behaviour, even though such perceptions may be erroneous. It is this acceptance of the importance of subjective reality which makes Rogers' position a phenomenological one. It means that it is not possible to fully understand another person unless one can appreciate the view that they have of themselves and the frame of reference in which they function. For example, I can only fully understand you and your actions if I interpret them in the light of your experience (probably unknown to me), values, attitudes and beliefs. However, I am far more likely to interpret your behaviour according to my own values, attitudes and beliefs. Consequently, I may not understand you at all, although I may claim to.

Ideal self

Not only is the 'self' concept important in Rogerian theory but also the 'ideal self'. This is the concept that one has of how one would really like to be, one which is highly valued. If one has a self-ideal which is unattainable one is on a fruitless journey. Most people are aware that they are different from the kind of person they would like to be, and in therapy there are indications that the ideal self may be modified, perhaps in the direction of a more realistic or achievable level. There is a greater congruence between the self and the ideal self.

A *holistic approach*

Another tenet of Rogerian theory is that personality is a holistic entity. It cannot be broken into segments for study or discussion. Alteration in any one part may produce change in another part. The individual (Rogers uses the term 'organism'), responds as a total being to events that are going on around him. 'The organism reacts as an organised whole to this phenomenal field'. (Rogers, 1951). For him the simple S–R type of explanation of behaviour seems almost impossible as the individual is then studied as an atomistic or segmental being.

Motivation

Contrary to Maslow's theory, Rogers proposes that there is only one motivating drive. It is a basic tendency human beings have within them to maintain and enhance themselves which energises behaviour in the direction of the full development of inherent potentialities. He calls this the self-actualisation tendency and he believes it to be common to all living things. As the organism develops there is an increase in the capacity for differentiation, with greater independence and integration. This growth is clearly evident in the young child as he moves towards independence and self-responsibility, even though this process is often painful. If the organism's behaviour is to enhance itself then choice must be exercised. Activities which enhance one will be positively evaluated and therefore sought after, while those actions which do not maintain or enhance the organism will be avoided. The individual is considered to be free to choose in a responsible way what is best for him. The person who engages in art and sculpture, has positively evaluated these pursuits and seeks them in order to develop not only creativity, achievement and satisfaction but also to increase self-sufficiency and autonomy, all part of the actualising process.

Application

The nurturing environment

Like plants, each person grows well if nurtured in the most appropriate environment, and for people that environment must consist of acceptance, respect and love from significant others. It is Rogers' belief that the development of the well-adjusted person depends upon the individual receiving 'unconditional positive regard'. This is clearly seen in the young child's need for love and approval from parents when an excited five-year-old rushes in from school with the shout 'Look what we did today mummy', holding up a picture for mum to look at; and whether approval is given or not will have a very powerful effect upon the shaping of the child's self-concept. However, apart from parents, most other significant people in a person's life make positive regard conditional upon behaviour. Sometimes parents themselves do this without thinking. 'Mummy won't love you if you do not behave', is a statement I have heard when out shopping. Good behaviour elicits love and acceptance, i.e. positive regard, but bad behaviour results in threats of no love. What the child hears is that she is only loved if she is good. Conditions are applied to her acceptance as a being, which lead to a belief that one is not wholly worthy or of value, consequently the individual strives hard to behave in a way which is acceptable to others, rather than in a way which 'enhances the self'. This may lead to conflict and stress. In well-adjusted people both the 'self' and the 'organism' are initiating and controlling behaviour. When they work together in harmony there is consistency between the self and the experience of the organism. The experience one has of an event or incident fits easily into one's self-concept as being a particular type of person. There is no conflict, 'congruence' prevails. 'Incongruence' refers to a discrepancy between the self and the experience of the organism. I have a friend who, I believe, sees himself as an attractive, helpful, interesting gentle person, who insists when I meet him in telling me all about his past adventures, the successes he has had, the important people he knows, and the exotic places he has visited. His language style is slow, ponderous, rather pompous and full of 'I'. I am sure that my perception of him, and I have checked that I am not alone in thinking him a bore, bears no resemblance to his own self-concept. The messages I give non-verbally say one thing, what he percieves is another, for distortion occurs in the process. Reality is prevented from entering consciousness and he could be described in Rogerian terms as being in a state of incongruence. If a person becomes aware of this incongruence, behaviour can be changed to maintain self-concept or one might have to modify one's self-concept in the light of inconsistent behaviour. Experiences which are too threatening are denied awareness and Freudian-type defence mechanisms operate in order to maintain the integrity of the self.

Maladjusted behaviour

Excessive use of defence mechanisms results in 'neurotic' behaviour, because the individual's actual behaviour is too far out of step with his self-concept. As more and more experiences are denied awareness, the self loses touch with reality and the person becomes more and more maladjusted. He lives according to a preconceived plan rather than existentially; he cannot trust himself and feels manipulated rather than free. This creates tension, and if it becomes severe it may interfere in a person's life to such a degree that the whole personality disintegrates.

Requirements for change

For a person to become 'fully-functioning' again with an integrated personality, unconditional self-regard must increase and the conditions of worth that a person places himself under must be reduced. This is only likely to occur if the person receives unconditional positive regard from significant people in his life. This is not easy; it means accepting the individual, irrespective of his values and behaviour, just as he is. This will facilitate the growth of his own unconditional positive regard, a reduction of his defensive behaviour and encourage an opening of self to new life experiences which will enhance his being. This approach is the basis of Rogers' Client Centred Therapy. However, unconditional positive regard alone is not sufficient to induce change. Other qualities are recognised as being of great importance. These are warmth, genuiness (sincerity) and empathy, the ability to appreciate another person's point of view from their own standpoint. It means entering another person's private perceptual world, being sensitive to what is going on in that person without making judgements.

'To be with another in this way means that for the time being you lay aside the views and values you hold for yourself in order to enter another's world without prejudice. In some senses, it means that you lay aside yourself and this can only be done by a person who is secure enough in himself that he knows he will not get lost in what may turn out to be the strange or bizzare world of the other, and can comfortably return to his own world when he wishes.' (Rogers, 1975).

Rogers encourages researchers to study his approach and these three qualities have been found to be important for encouraging change.

Group work

In recent years Rogers has become more involved in Encounter Groups. He published a book under that heading in 1970. This extension of his activities does not in any way oppose his previous work, for small group work is based upon the same principles embedded in humanistic psychology. The aim is for individual members of the groups to drop their social 'fronts' and behave in a way more true to themselves, expressing feelings honestly and openly. This experience can be a highly emotional one and lead to confrontations. If the confrontations are resolved, and members are accepted for who they are, healing processes can begin. As in counselling, the individual hopefully will lower his conditions of worth, reduce defensive behaviour and develop a more realistic evaluation of the self which can be openly expressed as confidence grows. Again these processes are facilitated in an atmosphere of warmth, genuiness, empathy and unconditional positive regard. This is a method of treatment in which many occupational therapists are involved and will be expanded later in Chapter 9.

SUMMARY

It is clear that although Maslow and Rogers differ in many ways, they have a great deal in common. In general, humanistic psychologists have a great belief in the goodness of human nature. People have an innate drive to grow, create and love. They have the power to make choices through which they can direct their own lives. Healthy growth depends upon an environment providing the necessary prerequisites. If this occurs, the individual will develop his full genetic potential. Without the right environment the person's growth can be stunted; they may become aggressive, defensive and then develop maladjusted behaviour. The importance of the subjective experience in the humanistic tradition makes scientific study difficult; even so, some research has attempted to evaluate this approach as a means of change. More about this can be found in *Personality, Theory, Measurement and Research* edited by Fay Fransella (1982). This perspective keeps the individual as a total being at the centre of study, even where there is illness or psychological disturbance. Such processes are not considered in isolation from the person. It rightly earns the title a Person Centred Approach.

REFERENCES

Fransella F 1982 Psychology for occupational therapists. British Psychological Society in association with the Macmillan Press, London
Maslow A H 1954 Motivation and personality. Harper and Row, New York
Maslow A H 1968 Towards a psychology of being, D Van Nostrand Company, New York
May R 1953 Man's search for himself. New American Library (Signet), New York
Rogers C R 1951 Client centered therapy. Constable, London
Rogers C R 1959 A theory of therapy, personality and inter-personal relationships, as developed in the client centred framework. In Koch S (ed) Psychology; a study of science, Volume 3. McGraw-Hill, New York
Rogers C R 1975 Empathic: an unappreciated way of being. The Counselling Psychologist 3: 2
Rowan J 1976 Ordinary ecstasy: humanistic psychology in action. Routledge and Kegan Paul, London

Attitudes and attitudinal change

INTRODUCTION

If occupational therapy is rightly described as a social process then it is appropriate to lay stress on the attitudes which people hold and which direct their behaviour towards themselves, objects, ideas and others. The study of attitudes is a central theme within social psychology. However, this is also a subject which has interested a wide range of thinkers and writers over many decades. If you pick up a psychology textbook you will probably find attitudes stuck between cognition and social behaviour, and, perhaps, find little justification in its selection as a major topic here. If you pick up any other book, from shelves marked philosophy, politics, travel, fiction, poetry or even gardening, you will be bombarded by both the attitudes held by others and also a wide variety of attempts to describe the significance of attitudes and the circumstances of change. Because we have chosen to draw from a wide variety of sources, and not to depend on experimental psychology, it is important that the reader balances the material against study of individual disciplines including psychology and sociology. The right to be eclectic has to be earned.

Attitudes are an important influence on therapy because they affect, very profoundly, both the therapist and the client. They also determine, to a large extent, the relationship between these two. Individuals who choose to become occupational therapists do so for reasons which include certain beliefs about higher education, career structure, their own abilities and interests, the concept of service and the security of reasonably paid employment. Such an individual is also likely to value more abstract qualities such as the freedom and independence of the individual, self-fulfilment, courage and kindness. The changes in attitude which may be experienced by a student of occupational therapy, between enrolling on a course and qualifying, are in many cases predictable. Certain beliefs are acquired such as those concerning the effectiveness of some of the measures described in this book. Those values which are acknowledged by the profession as being appropriate to its practitioners are reinforced. This is not to say that the outcome is inevitable but those readers who are interested in the process of 'professionalisation' may care to pursue this subject further.

The client may find that his attitudes form part of the problem rather than being an inherent part of a successful biography. He may also find that professional staff are requiring of him that he should change, either in terms of relatively minor adaptations or in very radical ways. His decision as to whether to make such changes or not, and his ability to change will be largely determined by the attitudes which he currently holds, their source, their strength and their validity.

There is a third reason for perceiving this topic to have some importance. Occupational therapists work as part of multidisciplinary teams within which the contribution, and the attitudes, of each member regulates the quality of care offered to the clients. Only by identifying attitudes, and appreciating the way in which they are formed and the influence that they have, can we coordinate our concerns and create an environment in which the clients' needs become the 'figure' and our own differences the 'ground'.

ATTITUDES

Difficulties of definition

In order to define an attitude it is necessary to recognise its components. Although there is some dissention about the boundary between these components most sources suggest that they number three. The two internal factors are beliefs, which are essentially to do with cognition, and values (or evaluations) which are to do with emotion. The third part is behaviour or action through which these internal factors are expressed. It follows that one cannot come to an understanding of what an attitude is without reference to beliefs and values. The changing of attitudes, and change in behaviour as an outward expression of attitude, is also reliant on understanding beliefs and values, how they have been formed in the past and from where they derive their strength.

Already this has begun to sound complicated. There is some fundamental controversy within social psychology over the definition of terms. It sometimes appears that the sementic battles supercede the research of the subject and totally satisfying definitions have rarely been attained. One may easily be confused by terms or have a blurred idea of the differences between them. Because attitudes, beliefs and values are 'loaded' topics, and because they are important to the individual, they are frequently bandied about. Perhaps they are rarely understood with clarity because they are accepted without question as an integral part of the self.

Historically, Allport in 1935 identified three points of origin of modern concepts about attitudes. These were:

1. In the experimental psychology of the late nineteenth century (which included the investigation of perception, judgement, thought and volition).
2. In psychoanalysis (which emphasised that attitudes had both dynamic and unconscious bases).
3. In sociology (which admitted underlying social and cultural influences).

Rokeach (1968) writing over thirty years later accepted this basic view but also mentions the enduring interest of both philosophers and theologians in the underlying dynamics. His own definition of attitude appears to be one of the clearest and the simplest from which to work: 'An attitude is a relatively enduring organisation of beliefs around an object or situation predisposing one to respond in some preferential manner'.

It is to the nature of beliefs and their organisation that we now turn, in order to appreciate the way in which attitudes are created.

Beliefs

Individuals possess an enormous number of beliefs. These have a degree of connection and interdependence which causes them to be organised into 'belief systems'. These have their consequences in the way individuals behave, the expressive or active component of attitudes. Beliefs are not always immediately apparent. Social and personal factors often impinge upon them and this means that they must often be inferred.

Systems of beliefs can be viewed as part of the architecture of the personality. Certain beliefs can be said to be central to the individual; these also have connections with other peripheral beliefs. They are rather like the central columns which hold up a building; they are vital to its perceived structure with other less fundamental 'pillars' outlying and complementing them. The result is a hopefully harmonious edifice which will be unique to each person, although the general method of construction or formation is similar. Central beliefs, because of their nucleic nature, are far harder to change than peripheral beliefs. This latter type tend to bear less relation to each other and 'splitting' them is far less likely to threaten the overall structure.

According to Rokeach, types of belief can be categorised in terms of their centrality to the individual who holds them.

1. Primary beliefs to do with existence

This concept deals with the central and essential beliefs held by an individual. They form the cornerstone of the structure and have the greatest connection with other beliefs. The fundamental nature of these beliefs concerns one's own existence and identity in the physical and social world. Simple examples might include:

'I know that my name is _____'
'I know that I have two legs'

2. Shared and unshared primary beliefs

The group of beliefs above may or may not be held in common with other people. Those which are shared, and presumably therefore reinforced, are said to have greater centrality and to be more connected with other beliefs than primary beliefs which are unshared. An example of a shared belief might be:

'I know that the world is round'
An example of an unshared belief might be:
'I know that I have unrecognised artistic ability'

3. Those of direct or indirect source

Rokeach points out that some beliefs are underived, that is they arise out of direct encounter with the object and others are derived through contact with some person or authority. An example of an underived belief might be:

'I know, having met Mrs Smith, that she has one grey eye and one green eye'
A derived belief may have the same content but has been obtained through contact with an intermediary. Hence:

'I know, from talking to Mrs Drinkwater that Mrs Smith has one grey and one green eye'.

Because of the distance between the individual and the object of his belief it will hold a weaker position in the connecting system than an underived belief.

4. Beliefs concerning taste

Many beliefs fall into this category. They concern arbitrary matters of taste and are relevant only to the person who holds these beliefs. For example:

'I know that I enjoy Mozart's music and I believe him to be one of the world's greatest composers'.

This type of belief is said to have little connection or consequence within the system of beliefs compared with those not concerning arbitrary matters of taste.

Having established that beliefs can vary in their centrality to the individual we can now examine why some beliefs are less moveable than others.

The beliefs concerned with existence form the inner core of an individual's system of beliefs. These beliefs may be shared with others and are so primary that they are rarely confronted. When a shared belief ceases to be held in common with others then the individual is called upon to examine the validity of his own senses, and possibly even his sanity.

The majority of people, for example, share the belief that the earth is round. It may be shown to us as a flattened rectangle or as a number of segments in a printed atlas. However, we believe in its roundness despite these distortions. There are a number of reasons for this belief. First of all, shared realities have been built up from childhood through the influence of parents or other significant people. Your mother and father *told* you that the earth is round and you believed them. The beliefs arising from many of such shared realities become an integral part of the individual's belief system. Here we have an obvious cross-link with sociology, in particular the role of primary socialization. Part of believing the earth to be round stems from believing an authority. In other words, having seen pictures of the spherical earth on the television or in newspapers we believe it is round because we believe in the authority that says so.

White (1959) described how the violation of a *central* belief leads to disturbance of beliefs concerning self-identity and the ability to function competently. Imagine the disruption of a central belief as the hub of a seismic disturbance. The waves radiate out to connecting beliefs causing a threat to the entire structure. The individual then faces the painful, and painstaking, task of reconstruction. A therapist who is concerned with those who have found bereavement too great a trauma to recover from unaided may find this a useful concept.

Certain primary beliefs result from interaction with the object of belief. These are not necessarily shared with others but become constant in the light of experience. Beliefs held in pure faith fall into this category and are relatively immoveable, for example:

'I believe in God . . .'

'I believe in the inherent goodness of mankind'

Non-primary beliefs also begin to emerge in childhood. They are less stable, expect to be contradicted, are not necessarily shared in common and are therefore more open to change. A child's belief in an imaginary friend may fall into this category.

The retention or rejection of these beliefs depends upon the person to whom the child refers for information or knowledge. Ultimately, the child compromises so that he perceives, and hence believes about the world, as rationally as his current maturity allows. At the same time he adjusts his beliefs so that they are as defensive and irrational as circumstances require. This may be seen as a sort of slide rule of belief which the child uses to cope with his rapidly changing self and environment.

Those beliefs which are derived originate from symbols of authority. The central belief is in the authority which could be a newspaper, a politician, a teacher or a therapist. The individual comes to believe in many of that authority's beliefs. I might, for example, believe in the political authority of the Mombanista Liberation Front. The members of the front believe, amongst other things, that vegetarianism is healthy and that government should be by proportional representation: I believe in both of these. My belief is partly due to a desire to be a member of the group and to be recognised by my fellow members. However, the possibility of ceasing to believe in the authority of the Mombanista Liberation Front implies mutability in my beliefs about vegetarianism and proportional representation.

'Belief systems' involve all the types of belief mentioned so far and it should begin to be possible to appreciate the tones and intensities of some beliefs over others. The ways in which each are flavoured by class, through parental influence and the desire to belong to specific social groups, are all part of the pattern of how comparable individuals acquire their own unique system.

Congruence of beliefs

Belief congruence needs to be considered in conjunction with systems of belief. Congruence relates to the way in which we measure, and sometimes assume, the beliefs of others on the basis of social relationships. Our own beliefs may be changed or retained as a result of our interaction with individuals or with groups.

The fact that one values the beliefs and the attitudes of others in proportion to their similarity to one's own has some bearing on the formation of social groupings. The attitudes of group members are identifiable, indeed almost predictable. For example, and at the risk of generalisation, those people who oppose nuclear defence systems are often those who oppose censorship and who hold ideals about greater social equality.

Any stimulus, a word, perception or event, may activate the relevant portion of a belief system. The spectrum of beliefs activated depends upon the impact and the breadth of the stimulus. For example, the word 'ecology' is more likely to have a broader impact on my belief systems than the words 'chemical fertiliser'. Thus, the individual will assess the importance of a given stimulus through his awareness of the beliefs it activates along the continuum of his own system of belief/disbelief and similarity/dissimilarity.

To relieve any tedium experienced in having to assimilate this theoretical background, try a practical exercise. Select a person known to you, who is at present receiving treatment for a psychiatric disorder, and hazard a guess at the following questions:

1. What beliefs do you know him to hold?
2. What beliefs do you think that he probably holds, even though these have not been expressed to your knowledge?
3. Do you associate his beliefs with his psychological problems, his social class or with his membership of any particular group (e.g. psychiatric patient, artist, humourist, social worker)?
4. Would it benefit him to change his beliefs?
5. To what extent have you answered the preceding questions through knowledge and to what extent through prejudice, assumption and through the bias that is a part of your own membership of certain groups?

Values

When we say that we value a friend or that we value our independence or freedom we are expressing something subtly different from a belief. To hold that courage or gentleness are desirable attributes or that lying or stealing are wrong, is to hold values. These have an emotional basis; they are about what we feel rather than what we think. They are also very powerful directors of action.

Values are acquired in ways similar to those in which a system of beliefs is built. Piaget (1965) and Kohlberg (1973) have both produced studies of the development of moral judgement in children. Although values are essentially an affective component, the ability to apply them to situations is developed in parallel with cognitive ability, if only because they involve the mastery of abstract concepts.

The simplest values are those which express fairly trivial likes or dislikes. I hate rice pudding: this doesn't mean that I believe rice pudding to be wrong or that I am concerned by the politics of rice production in the Third World, or that I was attacked by an enraged rice pudding in early childhood. I just hate rice pudding.

More significant likes and dislikes, which have a greater impact on attitudes and actions, are those which are directed towards social groups. These may include, for example, homosexuals, political parties, coloured immigrants, students or even entire nations. Even on a little group of islands, the British Isles, the English, the Scots, the Welsh and the Irish all apply values when generalising about each other, despite centuries of cheerful intermarriage.

Ideas about right and wrong are acquired throughout childhood and applied with varying degrees of maturity to the dilemmas of adult life. Maturity is a significant factor because, although two people may appear to hold a value in common, the underlying feelings about it might be different. For example two people may agree that it is wrong to remove office stationery for personal use. One may feel it's wrong because he might get caught and disciplined and the other because he feels that to act dishonestly is to confront his own integrity.

When we apply value judgements, those that involve discrimination between good/bad, right/wrong, pleasurable/unpleasant, to certain situations a degree of conflict can result. Take, for example, the general subjects of sex and of aggression. These two have in common that they are frequently subject to impulses and to very immediate emotional factors in the environment. Social convention requires that an individual should control the drives associated with each. It is interesting that a great many values are associated with these (many of which specify 'wrong' actions) and that violation of these values is particularly likely to lead to experiences of guilt.

Values mediate not only the actions of an individual but also help him to interpret the actions of others. They form a sounding board against which one can judge and justify ones own attitudes and actions or those of others. They also allow us to compare ourselves, favourably or unfavourably with others.

The dilemmas presented by life are usually a great deal more complicated than whether to steal stationery from the office or not. Much of our time is spent in discussing issues such as the abortion of abnormal foetuses, the concept of punishment, the right to take one's own life, the maintenance of confidentiality, the custody of children within failing marriages, vivisection and a hundred others. We bring both our values and our beliefs to such discussion, sometimes determined to maintain them and sometimes open to change or compromise. Values that are deeply held are as difficult to change as are central beliefs; in fact these two are often intimately related. Views are opposed as to whether a central core of values give rise to the system of beliefs or whether one's beliefs shape one's values. To attempt to unscramble this one is an interesting intellectual exercise but perhaps not essential here. That values are separate from beliefs is perhaps best illustrated by noting that values and moral judgements are an important topic in another discipline, philosophy. Jeremy Bentham (1748–1831) and John Stuart Mill (1806–1873) developed the 'Greatest Happiness Principle' as fundamental to their own version of Utilitarianism. Utilitarianism in this context is the doctrine which says that actions can be defined as being right or wrong according to their good or bad consequences. This cuts straight across some of the dilemmas raised within the topics mentioned above and suggests that the answer should always lie in the course of action which makes the most people happy, or at least causes suffering to the fewest. Applying this principle has some problems; it could for example lead a group of oppressed occupational therapy students to throw their tutor out of a fifth floor window. What would stop them would not be the sixth commandment but the long term unhappiness caused to them and their families during their imprisonment. The importance of introducing this topic here is not in suggesting it as a guiding principle for professional practice. It is an example of a fascinating attempt to organise the multitude of values which may conflict with one another, or create rather than resolve dilemmas, into a single dimension.

To return to the notion that an understanding of values is significant to occupational therapists, consider the client who has difficulty in applying values to his own behaviour. Bandura and Walters (1969) suggest that 'During the course of traditional therapy the client is exposed to many incidental cues involving the therapist's values, attitudes and patterns of behaviour. They are incidental only because they are usually considered secondary or irrelevant to the task of resolving the client's problems. Nevertheless, some of the changes observed in the client's behaviour may result, not so much from the intentional interaction between the client and the therapist, as from the active learning by the client of the therapist's attitudes and values that the therapist has not directly attempted to teach.' This comment is made in the light of studies indicating that the modification of values in relation to sex, aggression and authority, so that they approximate more closely to values held by the therapist, tends to be echoed by improvement in behaviour. Ideas such as this move the discussion on into the text section to examine the relevance of attitudes within education and practice.

The relevance of attitude

It is suggested, but not proven, that the attitudes held by an individual determine his behaviour. We can certainly assume that they have a very strong influence even though examples occur all the time of ourselves and others acting in unexpected ways. Given that this is a disturbed world in which people often fail to act in accordance with their expressed beliefs and attitudes, it is still much easier to predict what someone will do if we know what they think and feel about any given situation. It should also be possible to predict from a person's intentional behaviour which attitudes or relevant values he holds. In believing that we can contribute usefully to the assessment of an individual, through observation of him in different settings, we are already making an assumption that this is true. We talk about the attitudes of those in our care and consider them to be a significant factor in determining the success of therapy. This comment is made in relation to subjective assessment of attitudes and does not relate to formal attempts to measure attitudes such as those described by Oppenheim (1966).

The beliefs that a patient has, and the values which have significance to him may be a part of the problem for which he is receiving treatment. Cognitive dissonance, the discomfort experienced when one's beliefs and one's actions or desires are at variance, is described later in this chapter. This may be a common problem to those who are unable to cope normally and may give rise to depression or anxiety. Conversely the presence of emotional disturbance may create functional problems or a sufficient degree of doubts about the self that cognitive dissonance is created.

For other psychologically disturbed people there may be a primary disturbance of beliefs. Delusions were described within Chapter 1 as a form of cognitive abnormality. If someone does hold such false beliefs that cannot be shared with others then his entire structure of beliefs will not just be threatened but will be distorted. If we refer again to the simile of an architectural edifice such distortion would be like viewing the building through moving water.

The majority of patients hold beliefs about themselves or about reality that are not shared with others. These may be bizarre, may be related to specific features such as body image or may be generally applied to their own inadequacy, unworthiness or fear. The problem that faces a therapist lies in deciding whether to try to share these beliefs, thus reinforcing them but assisting the development of a personal relationship through empathy, or to contradict them. Contradiction may isolate the patient further but may provide a normal model of widely accepted beliefs. Probably the answer in many cases is to acknowledge the difference in beliefs held by both parties but not to introduce value judgements. This means that in offering a different point of view it is unwise to imply in any way that the other is wrong, bad or even silly. This sounds easy but how many of us have responded to someone who has expressed that they are loathsome in some way by countering 'Don't be silly, of course you are good and nice to know.'

We are now beginning to refer to the attitudes held by therapists and applied to the problems of others. It has already been noted that the holding of certain attitudes facilitates entry into social groups and maintains membership and status within these groups. The adoption of attitudes, or the emphasis placed on existing and relevant ones, is not a conscious process. In fact, the first time that someone claims to know that you are an occupational therapist because of your attitudes is often an occasion for offence. However, one can guard against being associated with attitudes which are offered to you as a short cut in thinking and evaluating for yourself.

Whilst talking to a group of medical students a psychiatrist was heard to say of alcoholics that 'they all smoke and they all tell lies'. This is an interesting statement, not because it adds to our clinical knowledge of alcoholism but because it reveals information about the attitudes of the speaker and how these may be transmitted to future members of the same professional group. Even though the observation was probably humorous we need to interpret it in terms of values held by the speaker. If he holds that both smoking and lying are 'bad' then is he implying that alcoholics are also 'bad'? If he is offering this as a personal value statement do the students recognise it as such or do they accept it as a belief? It would be interesting to know how many of them wrote it down and thus had this statement available to them at a later date, out of context, but recognisably arising from a source of authority.

Most students of occupational therapy have, like other students, some critical awareness of the values and beliefs of those who teach them, both in colleges and in clinical settings. Just as your own attitudes help you to interpret and to respond to the world so the appreciation of those held by others help you to mediate your experience of what they say and do. How much knowledge though should therapists have of their own attitudes and the way in which these affect the experience of the patient?

Like every other member of staff an occupational therapist models behaviour and models attitudes. It is not enough to realise that the client group knows whether or not you misuse health service time, materials, telephones or relationships. A complete range of beliefs, values and ways of interpreting these through behaviour are made available to those in receipt of therapy. If you are unaware of how all of these are represented within your self and your way of working then you probably have a poor idea of the environment which you create.

The next part of this chapter deals with the way in which change may be brought about. Whether changes in attitudes precede the ability to change one's behaviour, or whether change in behaviour can influence current attitudes is a natural line of enquiry for a therapist. In reading the material keep this question in mind.

CHANGE

Occupational therapists, even those employing behavioural techniques, do not 'change' people. Individuals can acquire different ideas and different patterns of behaviour through changes which are made in their environment but profound change comes from within. This second major section will review several of the more important topics within the whole subject of change. When individuals are living through an unstable period during which change is imminent, being resisted or actually happening, they may become extra sensitive or vulnerable within existing relationships. A therapist who is attempting to be personally available at this time would be wise to consider some of the underlying dynamics of change.

Change and equilibrium

Change and equilibrium appear to have a complementary relationship. At any one time, in a particular facet of the personality, change may predominate until equilibrium is found. This then remains predominant until such time as another change becomes necessary. This can be described as the seeking of homeostasis; this being a feeling of comfort and wellbeing within the individual resulting from having achieved the ideal internal environment—or the optimal psychological equilibrium for the individual at that moment. This concept was developed during the 1920s by 'drive theorists' and expanded by Maslow (1972) in his hierarchy of needs (see Ch. 4). The relationship between change and equilibrium also involves motivation. This can be illustrated through the parallel of driving a car.

An individual driving a car along an unknown road must inevitably move forward, but as he does so he meets many hazards such as dangerous bends, traffic lights and pedestrians. In order to travel satisfactorily it is not enough that he is able to to switch on the ignition, grasp the wheel and put his foot on the accelerator. He must constantly shift and change both gears and steering in order to remain safe and to continue travelling. He is motivated to stay alive and to reach his destination; his capacity to utilise change and equilibrium enables him to do so.

One can see, through this example, that change and equilibrium may exist only for brief periods and be almost indivisible. It should reasonably follow that while equilibrium implies stability and homeostasis it may conversely involve the tension of preparedness for change. This sounds like a paradox and, indeed, it is one. Change, in matters more complex than the driving of a car, is neither an easy thing to do nor an easy concept to grasp. However, as Burke (1729–1797) said, 'a State without the means of some change is without the means of its conservation'. This may apply as well to the government of the self as to the government of a state.

By changing, or becoming different in some way, one is forced to view a temporary chaos within the self. The perception of a need to change may be accompanied by the same somatic signs that are associated with other forms of anxiety, for example sweating and disturbances of digestion. It can feel, to some people, as though some temporary mistral were buffetting body and mind, uprooting well ordered concepts and ways of being. The emotional experience of change is the well used theme of poets, Ted Hughes (1972) describes how '. . . wind weilded blade-light' until '. . . the hills had new places' and, using the familiar image of a house to denote being '. . . the house rang like some fine green goblet in the note that any second would shatter it.'

Now, this may sound rather a dramatic way to describe, for example, trying to change from being a smoker to a non-smoker. It is important, however, to remember that many people do experience great stress in coming to terms with fundamental changes. They may feel as though they are attempting to grasp and mould matter in order to achieve even momentary equilibrium.

Change, then, is a paradox. By becoming aware of, or by focussing on an area requiring change, fifty per cent of the battle is won. Those who adopt a Gestalt style of thinking, term this as focussing on a 'figure'; this means becoming aware of the dominant feature in the immediate environment rather than what is background or 'ground'. For example, in the 'here and now' within which I write, my thoughts recede more and more into the 'ground', as discomfort in neck and shoulders urgently demand to become the 'figure' upon which my attention is focussed. The need for change is recognised, in posture, choice of chair or habits. Whatever form the change takes it will allow my neck and shoulders to become 'ground' again and some other internal or external feature to become 'figure'.

To illustrate a slightly different type of awareness and change, imagine sitting in an airport departure lounge with a terror of flying. By allowing the fear to become the dominant figure one may change the situation by running away or by concentrating upon the fear intently, coming to know it and to view it in perspective. This second strategy allows the fear to be re-assimilated in an inevitably mutated form into the self.

The onus is on the individual, indeed, if change is to be deep, and personal responsibility for it cannot be claimed by another person. Profound change must penetrate to the primary belief systems which, it will be remembered, are known often only to the individual. Hence, although change can be prompted from outside, the desire to change must come from within. Only you can hope to know yourself fully and therefore only you can hope to change that self. To examine this idea further, return to the example of the airport departure lounge. Only I know that my fear stems from a largely unshared belief that aeroplanes are far too heavy to fly and only remain in the air by chance. I conceived this belief through the direct confrontation of my mind and aircraft, irrespective of the number of times that helpful friends have explained to me the principles of turbo-jet propulsion. This belief will remain until, for the sake of my own comfort, I decide to look rationally at flight-safety statistics and to re-think turbo-jet propulsion. Then my attitude towards flying will stem from a better informed and more mature set of beliefs which allow me to consider flying to be actually possible, logical and safe.

Change appears to be as important within human groups as it is within individuals. Helmut Wilhelm stated: 'it is in constant change and growth alone that life can be grasped at all' and that 'to stand in the stream of this development is a datum of nature. To recognise it and follow it is responsibility and free choice'. Alfred Adler complemented this by saying, of change, that 'it is a goal seeking quality in the human soul . . .' that is continually '. . . seeking to map, plan, and direct its future towards a goal of security'. Security in this context may be equated with equilibrium.

To summarise briefly, it is necessary to be able to change in order to experience equilibrium. The ability to change requires a thorough knowledge of oneself, in effect a failure to change only occurs when an individual does not know and thoroughly accept all aspects of the self. By not having this knowledge and acceptance of himself an individual risks not experiencing the constant tide of change with every perception. In other words, he is not aware of what is taking place within himself and the delicate relationship between change and equilibrium breaks down. We can all recognise some of the dynamics as they occur in clients who cling rigidly to ways of thinking, feeling or responding, only to find that such resistance leads to anxiety or alienation rather than to security. Occupational therapists, their students and their teachers are not immune to these dangers, and one would be foolish to believe that they had less need to appreciate constant change and self appraisal.

The human task may be likened to that of attempting to ride a bicycle. One attempts to overcome disequilibria, by shifting and changing this way and that and by occupying and then voiding aspects of space. When the relationship between change and equilibrium breaks down then one risks falling off. Whilst learning how to maintain control there will be first gross and then fine 'wobbles' but once a sense of balance has been acquired then it is possible to get from place to place.

The danger of equilibrium is in the possibility of it becoming static. Changed sets of perceptions have a power that includes satisfaction to the individual who has found them (hence the dogmatism of the newly converted). Their initial impact risks them becoming calcified into patterns which resist further change. Perhaps one should attempt to regard change, self-awareness and equilibrium less as new and improved bricks and mortar, which sooner or later will impinge on vision, than as a vehicle for the fluidity and growth of ideas which will carry the individual forward. Learning to relinquish oneself into this flow may be seen as the achievement of true, and utterly simple, freedom.

Cognitive dissonance

The theory of cognitive dissonance explains in part how behaviour may influence attitudes and was described by Leon Festinger in 1957. 'Two cognitions that are inconsistant with one another will produce discomfort that motivates the person to remove the inconsistency and bring the cognitions into harmony'.

Indeed the dissonance experienced may be likened to the discomfort one experiences in playing or singing a dissonant note out of keeping with the general harmony of a piece of music. In life as in music, one invariably attempts to dispel the incongruity and to get it right next time.

The theory refers to conflicts which arise when the individual is faced with choices involving various cognitive elements. Festinger refers to these as 'knowledges'. This rather global term encompasses beliefs, values and attitudes. The 'knowledges' referred to may be seen as the currency of cognitive transactions—in finance as in cognition the result will sometimes be change.

Choices, conflicts and decisions arise in every area of life. Some choices involve a minimal degree of conflict while others involve the changing of an attitude or more fundamentally a belief. This process occurs in order to reduce the discomfort of the cognitive dissonance aroused by being faced with choice or decision.

The degree of dissonance felt depends partly on the importance of the cognitive elements or 'knowledges' involved and partly on the number of dissonant elements.

For example, a well-paid uninformed smoker who is only aware that his habit places a mild strain on his budget will experience far less cognitive dissonance in continuing to smoke than will a poorly-paid individual possessing many cognitive elements detailing the dangers to his health of continuing the habit.

Having experienced dissonance, the individual is driven to reduce it one of three ways.

1. Changing a behavioural cognitive element

For example, an overweight unfit man is informed of a family history of coronary heart disease, and is made aware of the dangers of his lifestyle. He possesses a number of cognitive elements which produce dissonance and he may therefore change his behaviour by dieting and taking some exercise, thus experiencing a reduction in cognitive dissonance.

2. Changing an environmental cognitive element

One may use as an example a depressed woman living in a pleasant home with a loving spouse. She may, in fact feel that her home is dreadful, filthy and unpleasant and therefore experience cognitive dissonance. She may feel compelled to destroy her possessions, littering the house and rendering it as filthy and unpleasant in reality as it is in her emotional perceptions. This action may have the effect of reducing the original dissonance.

3. Adding new cognitive elements

A drinker may reduce the dissonance he feels on being made aware of his potential alcoholism by reading material praising the social benefits of drinking or giving evidence of the ameliorative effects of small amounts of alcohol.

Cognitive dissonance may arise after a decision has been made. In general, the greater the importance of a decision, the greater will be the potential for dissonance. For example less dissonance will be aroused by the choice between two similarly priced bottles of dry French wine than between two motor cars.

Degrees of dissonance are also influenced by the similarity of the choices. For example, less dissonance will be aroused by the choice between buying two books than in choosing to buy either a book or a ticket for the theatre.

Dissonance arising from making decisions may be resolved in four ways.

1. Revoking the decision

Imagine an individual who has been consistently unhappy in his job and who subsequently argues with a superior. This may motivate him to consider resigning. Having made the decision. he may receive new information, for example that his superior's wife left him last week. This may leave him with a feeling that he ought to revoke his decision although it returns him to his original conflict.

2. Increasing the attractiveness of the chosen alternative

This is fairly well illustrated by the phenomenon that it is often the owners of a particular new model of motor car who avidly read the literature about it and who notice advertisements which praise it.

3. Decreasing the attractiveness of the unchosen alternative

This is the converse of two above. I shall be going to Blackpool this year. In Greece the drains, the heat, the food and the men are all equally hazardous.

4. Establishing a cognitive overlap

Having made the choice between a visit to the theatre or to the cinema, one classifies the two possibilities, deciding that both are forms of entertainment.

Perhaps one of the most relevant aspects of dissonance theory is that degree of conflict which is aroused by compliance. Compliance may be to pressure occurring without, or prior to, a change within the self.

The subject of persuasion is dealt with later in this chapter but it is obviously relevant to mention dissonance in relation to compliance here.

The amount of dissonance felt by an individual depends upon the reward that brings about the new behaviour or opinion. Token economies are an example of the way in which this may work beneficially. However, it must be remembered that pressure to change may be so distressing to an individual or may produce such intolerable dissonance that the decision is revoked. Similarly, the individual may find ways to sufficiently reduce the dissonance caused by non-compliance so that attempts to enforce change are meaningless.

Persuasion

We have already seen how an individual may change his attitudes, values or beliefs through the processes of cognitive dissonance. This may occur either before or after a change in behaviour. It has also been stated that if change is to be deep and personal it must stem from within. As a therapist one is faced with the problem of knowing that self-determination is the most effective force in bringing about change but also knowing that persuasion may have to be used in some cases.

Persuasion is a form of social influence in which one individual attempts to effect a change in the behaviour or opinions of another (Stang & Wrightsman, 1981).

Carl Hovland et al (1959) in researching changes in attitude determined four important factors which influence how open to persuasion an individual may be. These are attention, comprehension, readiness to accept new information and the retention of the message. It is obviously important for a therapist to bear these factors in mind and to pitch information appropriately. Various factors concerning the therapist's own attitudes should also be borne in mind, these are:

a. That the therapist appears to be knowledgeable about the topic under consideration. The effectiveness of this is borne out by the success of those advertisements which use, for example, high ranking ex-police officials to substantiate the safety of a new make of tyre.

b. That a rapport is achieved between the therapist and the person who is to be persuaded to change. Some new beliefs may be embraced because of an individual's liking for a therapist (Berkowitz, 1980). One might, however, question a change which took place ostensibly on this basis alone.

c. That the therapist appears enthusiastic about, and interested in, the persuasive message. It is clearly important that the therapist does believe wholeheartedly in what she is doing and trying to do for any individual.

d. The therapist must be, and must be perceived to be, trustworthy. There are two components to this. One comprises dependability and reliability, including the consistency of the message. The other concerns motivation which must be altruistically oriented towards the good of the patient.

All this places considerable responsibility upon the therapist. In presuming to attempt to change another it is important to know oneself thoroughly and to consider carefully the factors mentioned above. It follows that it is also both fair and more effective to present, and to talk through, both sides of any argument when in discussion with a patient. The absence of explanation or the arousal of fear are both counter-effective in encouraging change, and will obviously conflict with the four factors mentioned above. Repeated exposure to a message appears to reinforce its content and to promote change. It must also be remembered that a change may not be immediately apparent. The individual, hopefully, will digest information that has been given and use it as a catalyst for personal change and growth within his own good time.

Effective techniques which involve persuasion include several of those described within the third section of this book. All these involve the expression by the therapist of positive expectations regarding change. This means that any therapist should be aware of the responsibilities involved and guard against either exploiting the patients or requiring unrealistic changes. Changes in beliefs or attitudes are unlikely to take place where there is excessive coercion or compensation. It is to be hoped that a therapist will be sensitive to this, and having presented a case for change will allow each individual to determine its wisdom for himself and to acquire new attitudes which enable him to cope with the subject under discussion.

REFERENCES

Allport G W 1935 Attitudes. In Murchison C (ed) A handbook of social psychology. Clark University Press, Worcester, Massachusetts
Bandura A, Walters R H 1963 Social learning and personality development. Holt, Rinehart and Winson, New York
Berkowitz L A 1980 Survey of social psychology. Holt, Rinehart and Winson, New York
Festinger L 1957 A theory of cognitive dissonance. Stanford University Press, Stanford (California)
Hovland C I et al 1959 Reconciling conflicting results derived from experimental and survey studies of attitude change. American Psychologist 14: 8–17
Hughes T 1982 Selected poems 1957–67. Faber and Faber, London
Insko C A 1967 Theories of attitude change. Meredith, New York
Kohlberg L 1973 Implications of developmental psychology for education: examples from moral development. Educational Psychologist 10: 2–14
Oppenheim A N 1966 Questionnaire design and attitude measurement. Heinemann, London
Piaget J 1965 The moral judgement of the child. Free Press, New York
Rokeach M 1968 Beliefs, attitudes and values. Jossey Books, San Francisco
Stang D J, Wrightsman L S 1981 Dictionary of social behaviour and social research methods. Brooks, Cole, Monterey, California

White 1959 Motivation reconsidered: the concept of confidence. Psychological Review 59: 66

RECOMMENDED READING

Atkinson R L, Atkinson R C, Hilgard E R 1983 Introduction to psychology, 8th edn. Harcourt Brace Jovanovich, New York

Burns R B 1980 Essential psychology. M T P Press, Lancaster

DiMatteo D R, DiNicola D D 1982 Achieving patient compliance. Pergamon Press, Oxford

Forgas J P 1981 Social cognition, perspectives on everyday understanding. Academic Press, London

Keisler C A, Collins D E, Miller N 1969 Attitude change. John Wiley, New York

Lemon N 1973 Attitudes and their measurement. Batsford, London

Medcof J, Roth R 1979 Approaches to psychology. Open University Press, Milton Keynes

Perls F S, Hefferline R, Goodman P 1951 Gestalt therapy. Penguin Books, Harmondsworth

Reich B, Adcock C 1976 Values, attitudes and behaviour change. Methuen, London

Strongman K T 1979 Psychology for the paramedical professions. Croom Helm, London

6 *Joan King*

Social competence

INTRODUCTION

All psychological theories of behaviour deal with personal relationships. Psychoanalytic theory, for example, concerns itself with the conflicts aroused in an individual as a result of his interactions with significant other people in the past and which lead to psychiatric disorder. Learning theory, on the other hand, concentrates its attention on the effects of faulty learning on a person's behaviour in response to environmental stimuli. Man is a social animal and unless a person chooses to be a hermit other people are part of these environmental stimuli. As social relationships have become more complicated and the structure of society more complex, so the study of social behaviour has been recognised as being essential to explain the satisfactory or unsatisfactory adaptation of man to his environment.

At first the child undergoes the process of primary and secondary socialisation during which he acquires a sex role orientation. Social learning takes place by exposure to others, as models, in a variety of settings, for example, at home or at school. Later as an adult, other social roles in interpersonal relationships are required, like those associated with marriage, work and leisure activities. The ability to deal effectively with social encounters of varying kinds is highly desirable and contributes, to a considerable degree, to the state of mental well-being, not just of the individual but also those with whom he comes into contact. Through the process of socialisation and social learning the individual learns to react to different social requirements in different ways. To be successful, this learning must be adaptive to the environment, as opposed to maladaptive. If maladaptive, the consequences may, if extreme, lead to mental ill-health.

Because the social competence is a desired form of behaviour, it is equally desirable to be able to distinguish its features and characteristics.

110

Recognition of social competence is relatively easy on a subjective level, but objective qualitative and quantitative assessment is just as important as an objective personality test which shows individual facets of personality. An important difference is that personality tests are carried out in asocial conditions, whereas social skills and social competence assessment can be undertaken in a real situation.

Harré and Secord (1972) define social competence as the sum of the features of a social situation in which the individual finds himself and has to cope. To illustrate the varying levels of social competence required for an identical event taking place in different settings, imagine two separate occasions in which eight people are seated at a table, eating corn on the cob and engaged in conversation at the same time. In the first instance those present are parents with three teenage children and three friends; it is lunchtime on Saturday, all are seated round the kitchen table. Compare this with an equivalent situation of host and hostess with two married couples and two other guests, one male, one female. The host knows two of the male guests well; his wife meets one of the married couples fairly regularly. Each guest is there as spouse or as a professional person, in his or her own right. What is going on is a formal dinner party. It is taking place in the residence of the First Secretary of the British Embassy in Buenos Aires.

The requisite social behaviour in each instance would be very different.

BEHAVIOURAL PROCESSES

There is perpetual debate amongst social psychologists of different theoretical standpoints, for example trait theorists on the one hand and behaviourists or social learning theorists on the other, as to whether variations in behaviour stem more from the personality of the individual than from the situation. In either case, however, peoples' perception of situations, coupled with their reactions to and behaviour in them, is usually described in terms of personality traits or attributes rather than situational ones.

The most recent, interactionist, school of thought may be seen to be a marriage of the other two, as it recognises that behaviour is a combined function of the person and the situation, with stability of behavioural traits being shown within the constraints imposed by that situation. In other words, the person *and* the situation are important, but neither can be assessed in isolation.

The complicated interplay of persons and situations in determining and describing interactional behaviour can be reduced, in simplified form, to four basic features (Magnusson, 1974):

1. The behaviour of the individual in a situation depends to some extent upon the characteristics of that situation.
2. The influence on the behaviour of an individual, in kind and degree, differs from situation to situation according to the characteristics of each situation.
3. The influence on the behaviour of an individual that a situation exerts in degree, varies from individual to individual.
4. The influence on the behaviour of an individual in a specific situation, in kind and degree, depends upon the meaning and significance that the individual attaches to it.

In the past, attention on behavioural processes has focussed on the variations resulting from personality characteristics, genetic endowment, cognitive aspects and environmental features. Until recently, less consideration has been given to the variables which arise from the situation itself. Those behavioural processes which have a significant effect on interactional encounters are described by Argyle, Furnham and Graham (1981) as aggression, altruism, assertiveness, attraction, conformity, gaze, leadership and self-disclosure.

Sources of aggression include those in the immediate physical environment, such as physical crowding in work or living conditions, prolonged exposure to heat, noise and the possibility of physical attack. More personal sources are derived from cultural norms (competitiveness), social learning or perceptual models (scenes of violence, real or imaginary).

Behaviour which is intended to be helpful to others and promote helpful reactions from others (altruism) is an area of study wherein the conditions under which people indulge in pro-social acts has been given as much attention as the personalities involved. Also, more observation and experimentation has been undertaken in natural settings than in other investigations of social competence skills. The more familiar people are with a situation, the more likely they are to help; uncertainty leads to anxiety and apprehension. For example, a visitor may be reluctant to cook a meal in a friend's house if he is unfamiliar with a micro-wave oven, or is confused by a variety of verbal, written and practical instructions for its operation. Altruistic behaviour is inhibited in the presence of onlookers, although watching someone else helping makes one more likely to do so oneself.

In the United States social inadequacy is equated with lack of assertiveness, whereas in Britain the formation of friendships and interpersonal attraction are considered to be strongly indicative of social adequacy.

Friendship and interpersonal attraction do not happen as a matter of course. It is not enough to be compatible with, or complement, another's personality, attitudes, intellectual capabilities, social class etc. Similarities may strengthen friendship, but not necessarily lay its foundations nor guarantee it lasts. Physical attractiveness may affect attraction in brief encounters, but not exert the same effect in long-term relationships. Interpersonal attraction is subject to fluctuations, changes and developments over time. The social context in which it occurs also has a bearing on these episodic occurrences. Uncomfortable environmental conditions such as heat or noise can affect the degree to which we like or dislike others. According to our emotional state (happy, sad) strangers may be more or less atrractive to us.

Physical proximity both at home and at work can be either a positive or negative factor in the formation of friendships. If people are attracted to one another they will increase the number of times they meet and reduce the interval between them. Conversely, if people are not attracted from the start, they will reduce their encounters in number and length of time to the point where they ignore one another.

Much work remains to be done on the keeping of friends and the degree of intimacy that is shown in the structure or lack of structure we provide when we entertain our friends and acquaintances.

One of the behaviours most commonly encouraged and practised in occupational therapy is conformity, rooted as it is in receptiveness and persuasion by others and by social influences, such as social desirability. The sick person's level of social competence is invariably affected, and he is likely to experience difficulty in coping with, and readjusting to, change resulting from temporary or permanent disablement.

Gaze as a measure of social competence varies according to the amount of cooperation or affiliation which exists between people; where it is high it is increased. Those who like one another are more likely to look at one another. The greater the distance separating people in a room the more often they look at one another. Except when people are angry or pleading with others, they look less when talking about personal, than impersonal matters. A person held in high esteem, by status or leadership, for example, is likely to be looked at more by those of lesser standing.

It is found that gaze among people is reduced if objects or items are present which are of shared interest, which may be an argument for a balance of practical task groups and non-practical ones in occupational therapy.

'Appropriateness' is the most important feature of self-disclosure. If it is not appropriate in content (kind and amount), given at an opportune time, to the right recipients, it will be ineffectual. Most self-disclosure happens in groups of four people, of equal status, attractiveness, same sex, in private rather than in public.

ANALYSIS OF SOCIAL SITUATIONS

There is a need both for individual differences and for social situations to be analysed so that the difficulties people experience may be identified and methods of tackling the problem developed. Such methods have obvious application in a treatment situation. As in other settings used by occupational therapists, those for dealing with difficulties in social competence should resemble as closely as possible the real setting in which the social encounter or interaction which gives rise to difficulty would normally take place. Ideally, the best place to practise a skill is the natural one. However, some skills are practised in a variety of settings so that people are able to recognise the appropriateness of different skill in different conditions. A useful analogy may be that of learning to drive a car. At the outset it may be sensible to make use of a disused airfield for this purpose, whilst learning to synchronise clutch control with accelerator control, gear change with engine speed and so on. Subsequently, a car must be driven on the highway, in different traffic conditions and in different weather conditions before a skilled response is evoked on each occasion which produces minimal environmental risk to all concerned. A 'games' model is sometimes referred to in this respect (Argyle et al, 1981). Any game has a motivational structure which is functional in that certain goals must be met (viz, winning or not losing).

In the same way people in social situations aim to attain goals or subgoals which must be understood within the context of that situation. Social situations are structured in such a way that there may be a main goal but subsidiary goals as well. For example, the most important goal for an occupational therapist in relation to a patient, should be 'to ensure the highest level of coping in the other'.

'Looking after self' would be a secondary, or subsidiary goal to the main goal, as would 'earning a living'. As most social situations are likely to confront the person with two or more goals, conflicts may arise which will be discussed later in the chapter.

Social rules

We may be familiar with, if not practised in, one of the social rules of Tibet which requires a guest to belch to show appreciation of a meal; or alternatively we may know that a desert host is obliged to offer the greatest delicacy of the dish, sheeps' eyes, to the guest of honour. The rules of social behaviour are common to a culture or subculture and govern what behaviour may be deemed to be acceptable or unacceptable in any given situation. Such rules have evolved so that behaviour is regulated and coordinated for various goals to be achieved. Thus it is important for the occupational therapist to have an understanding of which rules and conventions apply to specific situations as well as to know why that rule is important and when it operates to attain a goal.

Social roles

During the course of any one day we may be required to take on a number of roles, for example, mother, daughter, staff member, interviewer or hostess. Within any social situation we may take on several roles, each interdependent upon the other and each with expectations of the individual regarding his or her responsibilities towards the others. Role systems evolve from situations so that goals may be attained. Both the occupational therapist and the patient need therefore to be aware of the various roles occupied by those participating in social situations, and the role responsibilities required.

Sequences of behaviour

The elements of behaviour follow a sequence. Goals or tasks are broken down into sub-goals or sub-tasks which have to be achieved or done in a particular order. Rituals and formal situations have a sequence of behaviour to be done in a special order. An interview follows a definite pattern: he who recognises the sequence in such a pattern is more likely to prove able in his behaviour to deal with it. This is analogous to making something from a construction kit, such as self-assembly kitchen cupboards, or making a dress from a paper pattern. Each is likely to fit together better and have a more professional finish if the instructions are followed in sequence. Sequences of behaviour help to distinguish what counts as a permissible role or rule from one which does not. It thus makes possible 'what happens now' and 'what happens next'.

Language and speech

Every group of people, whether it be of professionals, a family, or bounded by a geographical area, has its own 'language' such as accent, code, bilingualism. Similarly all social situations have particular features of the spoken word. These features are likely to be situation-specific. Some are restricted and constrained with regard to language use. Others call for modification in just one aspect of speech. 'Come along, my duck', may be acceptable from the bus conductor to a female passenger boarding a bus. It would not be acceptable from a stewardess to a businessman boarding a plane. Recognisably appropriate language must be learnt.

Stressful situations

Any social situation may potentially give rise to difficulty in coping or be a possible source of anxiety. Some situations, however, require a level of anxiety if they are to be managed effectively. The stress or anxiety may be experienced by the participant or perceived by others. Social difficulty is experienced when a person feels uncomfortable because he does not know what to do, or is embarrassed, or self-conscious. Stressful situations that are frequently met with produce in the person coping mechanisms which may be conscious or unconscious in order to reduce the anxiety of discomfort experienced.

Unease, difficulties and problems in social encounters are likely to be found as secondary or contributory features in psychiatric illness. They may be either causative in nature or arise as a result of psychiatric or physical disorder. Social competence has been found to be more important than formal psychiatric diagnosis in determining which people required hospitalisation and which were able to be maintained in the community (Gambrill, 1977).

Social needs

Twenty years after they first met, of Pippa an English woman, Sandy, her American friend and contemporary, said 'I don't know what it was, but she and I hit it off together right away': thus in a nutshell, an everyday acknowledgement that little is known about the mixture of behaviours which produce a mutually comfortable social situation. To feel comfortable a person needs to recognise social abilities in others and in themselves. Lack of social ability in themselves and others makes people experience discomfort. Being able to recognise and produce competent social behaviour is not sufficient in itself. There is also the need to understand the circumstances and the situations in which they are manifest.

DEFINITION OF SOCIAL COMPETENCE AND ASSERTIVENESS

It is difficult to define social competence, social skills, or assertiveness. Over sixteen definitions have been offered by various authorities which emphasise various different features. Some, particularly Americans, have chosen to define social competence exclusively in terms of assertiveness.

Three possible responses are provoked in situations requiring assertiveness: assertive, aggressive, or submissive behaviour.

Assertive behaviour is demonstrated by the individual who clearly, calmly and confidently explains to others by words or deeds his preferred line of action, with the result that others pay heed to what he says or does.

The aggressive individual on the other hand, uses speech or actions in an angry hostile fashion so that others 'give way', or 'give up' so that their views or rights in a situation are removed, rejected or ignored, thus enabling the aggressive person to attain his intended goals. He confronts others, denying them any options or choices.

The submissive person does not achieve his preferred aims because he allows others to make his decisions for him. He neither 'gives way' nor 'gives up' but 'gives in' passively to the wishes of others, along with the impression that he is wrong and others are right.

Assertiveness skills are those which are concerned with the search for, retention of, and improvement in, reinforcement of behaviour of self and others. These occur in social situations where the possibility also exists of loss of reinforcement or punishment. Four important features of assertiveness should be borne in mind:

(i) Where the assertion is positive, that is, the person takes the initiative, for example, in starting a conversation with others, or asking a favour.

(ii) Where the assertion is negative, that is the person takes the initiative in disagreeing with someone or admitting ignorance about some state of affairs.

(iii) Where the assertion is positive, but someone else takes the lead in initiating a conversation, or offers a compliment.

(iv) Where the assertion is negative in reply to someone else taking the initiative, for example in refusing a request.

Such distinctions are useful in assertiveness training as different reactions and replies will be needed in each of the four categories outlined. A person may be able to deal effectively with one category or situation, but may not manage, or deal with others equally satisfactorily or with the same degree of skill. Lack of generalisation of response strategies from one situation to another makes role play, which is discussed later in this chapter, a particularly useful means for assessment of assertiveness. A variety of situations can be set up and enacted to obtain as full a picture as possible of where weaknesses in assertiveness occur.

It is unusual for a person to be so socially unskilled as to have difficulty in dealing with all social situations, but most people are likely to experience varying degrees of discomfort, which may range from unease to anxiety in some settings. When two or more people are present in a situation (whether it be a task-oriented one, or a role-oriented one), a number of factors need to be considered about the effect they have on the social competence of those concerned. These are:

(i) The degree of intimacy involved

(ii) Whether the feelings expressed are positive or negative

(iii) Status, sex and age of the interactors

(iv) How the self is perceived in the situation

(v) How many people are present.

The following is an example of a task-oriented situation between shopkeeper and customer.

A middle-aged female customer, accompanied by friend of same age and sex, complains to a young woman behind the counter at a dry cleaners that one of a pair of her curtains has been torn whilst in their care. The customer is not satisfied with the explanations offered and asks to speak to the manager. Meanwhile, other customers have come into the shop, but remain unattended. The manager, a man in his late thirties, appears and gives his own possible reasons for the mishap, without either acknowledging or denying responsibility for what has happened. He eventually offers to have the curtain invisibly mended at the company's expense. The customer is not agreeable and wishes for compensation to the value of a new pair of curtains. The manager offers a sum of money which is below replacement cost and is unacceptable to the customer, who then introduces her friend as a member of a 'local consumer watchdog committee'. Full cash replacement is soon forthcoming, 'in the interests of good-will'.

The reader can readily imagine a scenario to fit an example of a role-oriented situation such as a session involving a small group of students and a member of staff. Similar, yet different, elements and factors affect the range of actions to be decided upon and carried out, and can be measured in terms of the social competence/incompetence shown. Some social psychologists, particularly Harré and Secord (1972), use a role-rule construct model for social behaviour, whereby they maintain that rules prompt or promote actions. These rules monitor and control performance, and this dramaturgical self-monitoring is a vital part of all social actions. In this manner, different 'personas' are presented which suit public or private occasions. They take the dramatic analogy further with the use of terms like scripts, entertainments and rituals.

SOCIAL DIFFICULTY

The discomfort and unease which the socially inadequate person feels produces a variety of reactions. These include anxiety, avoidance, anger, unhappiness, bewilderment and confusion.

Clinical and social psychologists have found that people seeking help to deal with their problems most commonly refer to the following as areas of difficulty:

(i) Intimacy: getting to know people, especially of the opposite sex; touching people.
(ii) Assertiveness: standing up for one's rights.
(iii) Being the centre of attention: having to 'perform' before others; for example, giving a talk, or being interviewed.
(iv) Social etiquette: correct behaviour in strange or unfamiliar settings.
(v) Fear of failure or rejection: lowering of, or damage to, self-esteem, confidence; for example, at a selection interview or taking a driving test.

(vi) Pain: even where the chance only exists; for example, a dental check-up, having an injection.

(vii) Separation and bereavement: stressful even if the separation is short-lived; for example, temporary absence overseas.

Other difficulties include assessment; for example getting a course assignment handed in on time, and rapid social change; for example, coming to terms with micro-technology.

If the past experience of the person has been that of physical or emotional pain or of social blundering and rejection, then he is likely either to avoid those situations in the future, or grow anxious in contemplation of future confrontations of a real or imagined kind (as in phobic states)?

It is clear, however, that the difficulties not only arise from the kind of person who finds himself in a *particular* situation, but also stem from the kind of situation a *particular* person finds himself in. It is not possible to generalise from person to person, nor from situation to situation.

It is important to identify the target behaviours to improve social competence. Improved ability to cope socially may be brought about by reducing the level of anxiety, as in behaviour therapy, or by social skills training (see Ch.). The individual's capabilities may also be enhanced by analysing and re-designing or re-engineering the situation which compounds the problem. An analogy may be that of motorway deterioration which is caused by constructional features and materials versus that produced by volume and density of traffic.

A situation becomes difficult if:

a. The motivation of the people in it, or the goals they seek are conflicting ones, or inappropriate to the various participants. For example a social gathering to celebrate an anniversary may also have as its aim the promotion, at work, of the host; interest in one's children by the headmaster of the local school; seeking professional advice; keeping the peace with difficult neighbours.

b. Rules are rigid or complicated, as can be seen in the order of protocol for serving food at an informal gathering at which civic dignitaries are present.

c. Self-confidence and skill are required to perform difficult assignments, such as standing in for an absent guest speaker.

d. There is no real previous experience of concepts related to particular situations, such as routine admission to hospital or attending court as a jury member.

ASSESSMENT METHODS

Just as there is no one definitive assessment test or method for measuring personality or intelligence, so it is with social competence. There are a number of techniques in use, each with its strengths and weaknesses. Neither has agreement been reached whether, for example, observed objective behaviour is better than self-reported behaviour or if a dimensional approach (using bi-polar scales and factor analysis) is preferable to a study of the elements of social competence (as in the 'games' theory referred to earlier). Yet other criticisms of the procedures used are that they are often culturally and situationally specific. Another factor is that the environmental setting in which the assessment is carried out may bear little comparison to the natural one in which the behaviour is, or should be, normally practised.

STRATEGIES FOR ASSESSMENT

The most common strategies used are:
1. Self report
2. Observational methods
3. Physiological measures.

1. Self-report methods

Commonly, these are (a) inventories or questionnaires (b) interviews and (c) self-monitoring techniques.

a. Inventories or questionnaires

These comprise items or statements whereof the person is asked to indicate how certain statements match his own behaviour, for example 'I often . . .', 'When . . . I sometimes . . .'. These provide a measure of assertiveness, social anxiety, or fear of disapproval. If given over a period of time, they are a useful source of information on how, and to what extent, a person perceives changes in his social behaviour, before, during and after training in areas of social skills deficits. Self-report tests like these, whilst easy to administer, in as much as the person can complete them unattended and in his own time, have a number of drawbacks. They are not especially useful with disturbed people, for example, the psychiatrically ill or newly-physically disabled, nor are they necessarily applicable to different age groups or those from varied socio-economic backgrounds. Secondly, there is no guarantee that the person can identify, recall and assess, with accuracy, how he behaved in another person's presence, or in a particular situation. Thirdly, he may not be able to distinguish clearly the behaviour of the other person in relation to himself. Hence, three kinds of perception are involved:

(i) interpersonal perception—perception of others
(ii) self-perception—perception of oneself in relation firstly to others, and secondly to the situation
(iii) meta-perception—the perception of other people's perception of oneself in an interpersonal exchange.

Each may be faulty. For example, can the individual discriminate that others are disapproving or that he is self-deprecatory. In self-report inventories which use comparative terms such as 'always', 'sometimes' or 'never', the respondent is obliged to make an indiscriminating 'usual', choice, that is to generalise about his behaviour; whereas, as has been shown earlier, the person who has no difficulty in refusing a shop assistant's 'Can I help you?', may seldom be able to say 'no' to a teenage daughter or son.

b. Interviews

These may be of the kind which prompt, or have a structure which encourages, information to be volunteered of a social interpersonal nature which depends upon the establishment of rapport. Most people describe their interpersonal lives in general, non-specific terms so that an interview should be structured to cover three phases of a person's life. Firstly, the retrospective phase, when the interviewee is asked about typical behavioural responses from childhood, for example did he behave in one way towards parents and in other to siblings and peers; was he hostile or shy when growing up. Another area of enquiry should be to discover how successfully common interpersonal tasks were mastered, such as the ability to handle 'give and take' situations with family, friends or spouse or the ability to resist pressure from others, to behave in an alien fashion. Secondly, the person should be asked about the present state of affairs, particularly with those he comes into most frequent contact, at home or at work. Thirdly, the interviewee should be asked to describe exactly what he says and does, both in verbal content and also in non-verbal behaviour (Eisler, 1978).

Joint interviews with interpersonal partners (spouse, close friends) also assist in revealing discrepancies in self-reported perception and how others perceive responses.

c. Self-monitoring techniques

This term is used when the person is asked to record his behaviour systematically and at prescribed intervals about how he presents himself both in his observable public behaviour and in private. This is usually done following a diary format. It has an advantage over other self-report methods as it provides and presents data that may not otherwise be readily accessible and which would be difficult to obtain by other means on a regular day-to-day basis. However, it does need to be used in conjunction with some independent monitoring to check the accuracy of the self-report. It is useful as a therapeutic tool because the measures of behaviour, self-assessed before treatment (assessment), are identical to those used to assess treatment (outcome). Also, the individual controls and 'grades' his own treatment to the extent that when he can recognise the frequency with which he behaves competently or incompetently, then he is able to instigate behaviour change for himself. Hence his rate of desirable or undesirable behaviour is likely to increase or decrease accordingly. It should be noted that one or two aspects of behaviour should be dealt with at a time, as the self-monitoring individual is only likely to be able to deal one or two target behaviours at once in a social situation.

2. Observational methods

These are (a) in vivo, (b) role play and (c) simulation.

a. In vivo

Because the multi-faceted, multidimensional complexities of social behaviour are demonstrated and recognised by overt responses, observation should be the assessment strategy of choice and 'in vivo' observation the most preferred. However, despite being the most realistic approach to pursue, it is also the least attainable, as it is difficult and expensive to realise in terms of personnel (trained observers), location (home, work, places of leisure) and recording methods (equipment). A number of interactions, for example positive/negative behaviour, conversational style and constant and problem-solving strategies used, can be investigated in this way, as well as ascertaining a person's response capability.

Other problems have arisen when this approach has been used with live observers or recording equipment. There is a tendency, when people are being directed and observed in performing common interpersonal activities to produce not their normal, but a 'better than average' response. Hence, there is a reaction to being observed, which distorts behaviour, so that the limits of the responses (effective or ineffective) may be assessed whilst the more customary behaviour patterns remain undisclosed. Also, much of the behaviour that observers would wish to witness occurs infrequently, unpredictably and out of sight, or off camera, so that the chances are slim of having the subject and the observer together at the right time and the right place.

b. Role play

This is the best known and most widely-used technique to observe behaviour, assess assertiveness and promote change. The basic format is that firstly an outline scenario is described to the individual. Then he is delivered an introductory cue line by another person, who behaves as if he were interacting in the scenario. The first individual then responds to the cue line, and a dialogue develops to role-playing the situation. In outline, this is the method normally used, although there are many variations, for example the use of pre-prepared, printed, or video-taped scenarios.

The role play should bear as close a resemblance to real life as possible with the circumstances leading up to the point at which the interaction begins, and its environmental context described with care. Additionally, the individual should be asked how he was feeling at the time and what he perceived the other person to be experiencing. In this way it is possible for both verbal and non-verbal behaviour to be assessed. Equal importance is placed on what the individual says, and how it is said, for example, on entering a room, or approaching another person. Props are best avoided or kept to a minimum as they may detract from or distort the interaction.

A variety of scenes or samples of behaviour in a number of situations should be collected, and role-played, to discover in how many, and in what kinds of contexts, behaviour may need to be altered to obtain the desired changes. It may be useful if the individual is asked by the other person to role-play his (the other person's) part first, to give that person an idea of how to behave in the role he is to assume. Alternatively, it may be feasible and useful to employ role-reversal as a technique.

Initially role play may be resisted, or thought unnatural by those undertaking it. This reaction is usually short-lived, when it is explained that it is a much more useful source of information than just talking about social incompetence or when one or two sessions have been completed.

c. Simulation

Naturalistic or 'as if' interaction is an alternative to role play in the assessment of social adequacy. It is a technique in which devised encounters are used which approximate to situations found in real life. People are presented with a variety of 'stage-managed' events to see how they respond to them as a measure of their assertiveness. Such 'rigged' situations can only take place if there is a considerable element of deception and collusion so that the individual is unaware of what is happening, and can be observed surreptitiously. Otherwise, the individual can be told what is happening and to behave 'as if' the interaction were real. As found with observational techniques, individuals perform better in an 'as if' setting, but acknowledge that their behaviour is more representative when the 'deception' method is used.

It is for such reasons that role play has advantages over other techniques, as it requires the individual to make quick and spontaneous replies from the outset of the interaction, and is useful to assess discrete responses. Simulation, on the other hand, is more suited to assess complex behaviour as it may last longer and allow the individual time to develop the role and maintain the interaction.

Although interaction using role play may elicit more anxiety in individuals, the use of videotape removes the individual one step away from real and direct confrontation with another person, as does the naturalistic or 'as if' simulation. The advantage, however, of the use of videotape, may lie in the fact that, during replay, attention can be drawn to different aspects of the social interaction and competency skills and on discrete responses such as the precise point or points when behaviour changes to become negative or positive. This might not otherwise be possible to note during a single observational session, or to replicate with accuracy during recall.

3. Physiological measures

The effects of arousal, negative and positive, on performance are well known, as are the physiological and physical accompaniments of anxiety. Objective measures of discomfort require laboratory conditions and techniques. These may be neither accessible or available, nor suited to social competency situations; nor may they be desirable in as much as they may induce or enhance a state of anxiety. Hence, most professionals rely upon an individual's subjective assessment of the degree of anxiety experienced. The same applies to arousal in the social situation whereby some assessment may be made of a self-report kind, in which the individual rates his level of anxiety over several familiar social situations, to determine his average rate of improvement as skill is increased.

FUTURE PROSPECTS

Social competence, like any other complex capability, is not acquired automatically, nor mastered exclusively as a result of some magical recipe in the correct proportions of the genetic, personality, intellectual, environmental and social endowments, of the individual. Every social interaction consists of a range of known elements, roles and rules, and has its accepted behavioural components. It elicits from the individual a series of responses, some negative and lacking in skill, some positive and effective. Each separate class or category of social interaction differs subtly from another. Much remains in theory to be learnt, and in practice to be solved, in the sphere of behaviour. However, as a theoretical and practical model, its future standing in both these areas is as assured as that of psychoanalysis, psychotherapy or other forms of personal or interpersonal counselling and treatment. It is a positive, educational, practical approach, which asserts that social competency may be learnt for the first time; where absent previously; relearnt where the initial, or previous learning experience has been inadequate or maladaptive or may be modified to meet the special needs of particular individuals/clients within any profession, such as orthopaedic surgeons, office staff, and occupational therapists alike.

REFERENCES

Argyle M, Furnham A, Graham J A 1981 Social situations. Cambridge University Press, Cambridge
Eisler R M 1978 The behavioural assessment of social skills. In: Hersen M, Bellack A S (eds) Behavioural assessment: a practical handbook. Pergamon, New York
Gambril E 1977 Behaviour modification. Jossey-Bass, San Francisco
Harre R, Secord P 1972 The explanation of social behaviour. Blackwell, Oxford
Magnusson D 1974 The individual in the situation: some studies of individuals' perceptions of situations. Stud. Psychol. 16: 124–132

RECOMMENDED READING

Argyle M 1978 The psychology of interpersonal behaviour, 3rd ed. Penguin, Harmondsworth
Ellis R, Whittington D 1983 New directions in social skills training. Croom Helm, London
Furnham A, King D J, Pendleton D 1980 Establishing rapport: interactional skills and occupational therapy. British Journal of Occupational Therapy 43: 322–325
Galassi M D, Galassi J P 1976 The effects of role playing variations on the assessment of assertive behaviour. Behavioural Therapy 7: 343–347
Johnson S M, Bolstad O D 1973 Methodological issues in naturalistic observation: some problems and solutions for field research. In: Hamerlynch L A, Hardy L C, Mash E J (eds) Behaviour change: methodology, concepts and practice. Research Press, Champaign, Illinois
Milgram S 1974 Obedience to authority. Harper and Row, New York
Pervin L A 1976 A free response description approach of person–situation interaction. Journal of personality and social psychology 34: 465–474
Trower P, Bryant B, Argyle M 1978 Social skills and mental health. Methuen, London

Practical intervention

Christine Hewitt

Training in social skills

INTRODUCTION

In recent years interest in the field of social skills has developed rapidly and training in social skills is now widespread. But the importance of socially skilled behaviour to the well-being of the individual is by no means a new discovery. Man is essentially a social animal. Throughout history the ability of the person to develop effective social skills and satisfying relationships with his fellows, has been one of his most significant accomplishments and attributes.

People need people. Society is made up of a network of relationships between people. If we take society to be like a large net, then the knots represent the people and the strands the communication between them. You cannot have a relationship without communication. An individual derives his greatest satisfaction in life through experiencing warm, positive and meaningful communication with others. Conversely, lack of communication or cold, deficient communication can affect a person's mental and physical health.

Communication skills are essential to the repertoire of social skills which each one of us employ in day to day living. Social skills include the use of verbal and non-verbal communication and a variety of specific social behaviours in given situations. Some people are less skilled in these social behaviours than others, but the term 'skill' (defined in the Oxford Dictionary as 'expertness, practised ability or facility in doing something') suggests that social skills may be learned and improved. This gives the whole notion of training in social skills a more positive and scientific basis.

THEORETICAL BASE

But before describing social skills and social skills training (or SST for short) in more detail, we need first to look at the theoretical rational upon which the learning of social skills is based. SST requires a specific approach as we shall see, but as a relatively new science it has a basis in other well-known theories. The values inherent in SST come principally from the humanistic approach found in the fields of education, applied psychology and psychotherapy. The methods adopted in SST are taken from the behavioural tradition of learning theory and training techniques.

Humanistic approach

Progressive educationalists such as Froebal (1887) have introduced the idea that the child is the person around whose needs all else should revolve and that learning relies on 'doing' and upon the child's inherent curiosity. This self-interest or motivation is echoed in the humanistic-existential approach to learning. For example, Carl Roger's (1965) 'Client-centred' or 'Non-directive' therapy, is seen as akin to good education and more fundamentally to the basic socialisation process. Roger's approach is client-centred in that he believes each person has a good human core and a self-help drive, so that people have both the inherent ability and motivation to change.

Another humanistic theorist, Maslow (1954) has helped to define this push towards growth or 'self-actualisation' in terms of a hierarchy of needs. These progress from the basic physiological needs such as hunger and thirst, through the cognitive needs, such as to know and understand, to the self-actualisation needs such as finding self-fulfilment and realising one's potential. The humanistic approach is much more positive and optimistic than, for example, Freud's psychoanalytical approach, because it emphasises that none of our innate needs is anti-social.

Thus we derive many of our values and goals from humanistic theories—and from psychotherapy we derive a basic format within which to train people in social skills. This is the 'self-help' group. Working with groups of individuals who share similar problems and who can help each other to solve them, is central to SST.

Behaviourist approach

The actual activity content of SST has been provided by another broad tradition, the behaviourist learning theories. Two important features are: that in the learning of skills, the skill or behavioural learning goal may be broken down into smaller more manageable parts. These can be learned separately and then put back together again into the more complex behaviour in question. For example, this occurs when we learn to drive a car. The skill of driving is broken down into smaller units of behaviour such as steering, changing gear and applying the brakes, which we learn separately, but eventually combine together to actually drive the car.

Social learning theory

The other important feature of behaviourism is in the concept of social learning. Bandura (1971) has developed a social learning theory which focusses on patterns of behaviour which are learned by the child as he grows up and which help him to cope with his environment. Learning takes place through the child modelling or imitating the behaviour of his parents, siblings, peers or teachers. This is reinforced in three ways. This may be directly by others, who may encourage or praise certain behaviours and discourage or ignore certain others. He will tend to learn and use more often the behaviours which are rewarded rather than those which are punished or ignored.

Reinforcement also takes place vicariously when the child observes the consequences of behaviour modelled by others. Self-reinforcement also develops when the child evaluates his own behaviour with self-praise or reproach, reward or punishment. Social learning theory emphasises the importance of the reciprocal interaction between the individual's behaviour and his environment and on the necessity to have adequate models. Children who are raised in isolation from other humans display socially unacceptable behaviour patterns. This is also found to be the case, although to a lesser extent, in children who are reared in a socially deprived home environment (Rutter, 1972)

Thus social learning theory combined with techniques of skills training and elements from other broad traditions, produce the values and methods for training in social skills. But what exactly are these social skills and how may they be acquired?

THE NATURE OF SOCIAL SKILLS

Many attempts have been made to define the terms 'social skills' and 'socially skilled'. Some of these definitions in general terms are 'communication skills', 'interaction skills' or 'social behaviour skills'. Some definitions are in terms of an ability. For example, 'the ability to interact with others in a given social context in specific ways that are socially accepted or valued and at the same time personally beneficial, mutually beneficial or beneficial primarily to others' (Combs & Slazby, 1937). And some definitions are in terms of behaviour. For example, Argyle (1981) describes socially skilled behaviour as 'social behaviour which is effective in realising the goals of the interactor'.

Another definition which seems to effectively combine the main aspects is—'a social skill is a set of goal-directed, inter-related social behaviours which can be learned and which are under the control of the individual' (Hargie et al, 1981).

This definition points out the distinction of the socially skilled person as having the ability to behave in an appropriate manner in a given situation. And it emphasises five main components of social skills:

1. Socially skilled behaviours are goal directed

The individual employs these behaviours knowingly as opposed to accidently, in order to achieve a specific purpose. For example, if A wishes to make friends with B, A will make eye-contact with B, nod, smile, move closer and engage B in conversation. Here, these behaviours are directed towards the goal of striking up a friendship.

2. Socially skilled behaviours should be inter-related

Each behaviour should be synchronised. As in the above example A should relate each behaviour to the goal of making friends, so that B will interpret each signal—the nod, the smile, as all relating to this goal. Thus, if each behaviour relates to the common goal, they are in this way inter-related and synchronised.

3. Social skills are defined in terms of identifiable units of behaviour

Social skills are learned in the same way as we learn motor skills such as riding a bicycle or baking a cake, that is, the whole skill is broken down into smaller more manageable units. Each one is learned separately and then integrated to form the larger unit of behaviour. Argyle (1972) argues that it is in this way, that an individual learns social skills. For example, the skill of making friends is comprised of a hierarchy of smaller elements, from making eye contact through to asking personal questions. An individual may be trained to acquire the smaller elements which will then build into the larger social response.

4. Social skills are comprised of behaviours which can be learned

The social learning theory (Bandura, 1971) applies in the learning of all social skills. As we have already discussed, this theory focuses on patterns of behaviour which are learned through coping with the environment. Learning is reinforced either directly or vicariously and cognitive processes enable the individual to anticipate possible consequences of his behaviour and thus change it accordingly. Self-reinforcement also motivates the individual to choose the most appropriate social response.

Thus an individual will learn through experience or may be taught which pattern of behaviours are most effective in making friends and will also learn to modify these behaviours in varying situations. For example, there will be some specific behaviours which are more appropraite when making friends with someone of the same sex, than with someone of the opposite sex.

5. Social skills should be under the control of the individual

This element of control may make the difference between a 'socially skilled' and a 'socially inadequate' person. The latter may have learned all the correct elements of social behaviours but be unable to organise and use them appropriately in given social situations. For example, the basic social skills required to form a friendship will be inappropriate if used by a jury member in a formal court hearing.

Social skills are relevant to everyday living and are used by each one of us from the moment we get up in the morning, to the moment we fall asleep. At the lowest level they include being able to dress ourselves through a spectrum of skills to the highest level, which involve making and maintaining close relationships with other people. So having looked at the nature of social skills in general, we now need to identify specific social skills.

Non-verbal and verbal communication

Social skills may be broadly divided into non-verbal communication (NVC for short) and verbal communication skills. Birdwhistell (1970) studied the relative importance of NVC to verbal communication and discovered that on average, out of a 24 hour period of leisure time, we speak for only about ten to eleven minutes. In addition only one-third of social meaning is carried by verbal communication, whilst two-thirds is carried by NVC, and may be nearer 90 per cent in some cases.

It is also interesting to note that verbally, women are better liars than men, but that non-verbally neither sex is able to lie. For example, verbally we may express love for another person, but if we do not really feel it, then our non-verbal behaviour will be contradictory. These non-verbal 'social leakages' may include avoiding eye contact or touch or leaning away from the person. Thus in the words of the song, 'it's not what she says but the way that she says it'!

Non-verbal communication also serves a number of important purposes, depending on the context in which it is used. According to Hargie et al (1981), most of these purposes are in relation to verbal communication. They are variously to replace, compliment, reinforce, emphasise or regulate the flow of verbal communication; or to initiate or sustain verbal communication or to influence other people's behaviour or to define acceptable patterns of behaviour.

Non-verbal communication

Hargie et al (1981) go on to list nine main forms of NVC. These are:
1. Bodily contact
2. Proximity
3. Orientation
4. Posture
5. Gestures and body movements
6. Facial expressions
7. Eye contact
8. Appearance
9. Paralanguage.

1. Bodily contact

This is our first experience of social communication, and experiments both with animals (Harlow 1966) and humans (Bowlby 1969), have shown that touch and close attachments at an early age (and especially to the mother) are crucial to subsequent healthy behavioural development. As the child grows up, touch contact is used between friends of the same and subsequently the opposite sex, mainly to establish and maintain relationships. During adult life there are certain taboos on both the amount and kind of bodily contact which is socially acceptable in given situations.

There are also a number of cultural differences. Jourard (1966) studied bodily contact in cafes all over the world. He discovered major cultural differences. For example, in Paris people would touch each other one hundred and twenty times in one hour, whilst in London in one hour, there would be no touching. However, there are also some cross-cultural norms in specific social situations, such as shaking hands or kissing when meeting or taking leave of someone.

In addition, a number of professionals touch in a certain way. For example, occupational therapists and their patients; hair-dressers and their clients. This kind of touching, however, is seen as a necessary function of that particular job and not as carrying the same connotations as other less 'professional' relations. But whatever the relationship, the important functions of touching between adults are to produce a feeling of intimacy and on a less intense level to show caring and concern and to give encouragement and support.

2. Proximity

Proximity has to do with the position, in terms of distance, that we take up when relating to one another. Hall (1959) defined distance into four main zones, depending on the purpose of the interaction.

The intimate zone (O to 18 inches) applies to those with intimate relationships, such as lovers.

The personal zone (18 inches to 4 feet) applies to those with close relationships, such as friends.

The social/consultative zone (4 feet to 12 feet) applies to those with less close or professional relationships, such as occupational therapists, doctors, teachers or solicitors (and who may relate from behind a desk).

The public zone (12 feet plus) applies to royalty, MPs or public speakers who are usually placed over 12 feet from their audience.

Thus the position we take up in a dyadic (one to one) or group (more than two) encounter, will have an effect on the kind of relationship we hope to achieve.

3. Orientation

This is linked with proximity and has to do with the angle of the whole body when relating to another and also to the seating arrangements. Side by side positioning indicates cooperation, whilst face to face is more competitive. Conversation seems to be most facilitated when chairs/people are at 90° to each other, and co-action is encouraged when chairs are placed on either side of a table, but not directly opposite. Spatial behaviour is connected with establishing territories. Personal space is that immediate space around a person which, if another person moves too close, becomes 'invaded'. Personal territory, however, is much larger and may be a person's desk area or own flat.

4. Posture

There are three main categories of human posture—standing, sitting or squatting and lying down. Posture can also affect the interaction between people. When both are either seated or standing, interaction is more prolonged and relaxed. If one is seated and one is standing, the relative positions may be threatening. Intense emotions, such as anxiety or depression can be picked up through a person's posture or body language.

5. Gestures and body movement

Friedman and Hoffman (1967) distinguish between gestures that are linked with speech and are directed towards objects or events as aids to communication, and gestures which are orientated towards self and are more to do with the release of tension. For example, among many gestures and body movements, we wave our hands when saying 'Goodbye' and we drum our fingers when impatient. 'Social leakage' occurs when the movements are unconscious, but unintentionally display otherwise hidden emotions. For example, fiddling with an ear lobe or earring may be a self-comforting gesture.

6. Facial expressions

Osgood (1966) has suggested that facial expression portrays seven main emotions: happiness, fear, sadness, anger, surprise, disgust/contempt and interest. The eyes and the mouth are two regions of the face which can express the most emotion although the eyebrows, lips and tongue are also utilised. Blushing is a 'social leakage' which can denote fear, anger or embarassment.

7. Eye contact

Eye contact or mutual gaze almost invariably initiates some kind of interaction, so is most important. After contact is made, the movements of the eyes control and synchronise the conversation. In a dyadic encounter the listener looks at the speaker twice as much and where there is a stronger emotional content in the inter-action, whether loving or angry, the eye contact will also be more intense.

8. Appearance

Physical appearance includes face, hair, body shape and clothes. Facial expression is, of course, very important, but so too is the appearance of the skin, whether it shows ageing or is made-up or not. Hair may also give clues about the person; short back and sides or long, dyed hair may indicate social grouping, as in the 'army', or a 'punk' hairstyle. Despite women's lib., it is still more accept-able in this country for women to be smaller and slimmer and for men to be taller and stronger. Clothes also tell us about a person, whether they are fashionable or conservative, brightly coloured or drab. Certain clothes or uniforms may tell us about a person's status, for example, hospital or school uniforms.

9. Paralanguage

Paralinguistics is commonly referred to as that which is left after sub-tracting the verbal content from speech. It is the vocal expression and includes the tone, pitch sound level and speed of vocal expression. Paralanguage conveys both emotional and factual infor-mation and adds emphasis to the spoken word. Thus it is very important. The same sentence 'John is giving me his pen' may have separate meanings, depending upon which word the emphasis is placed. Paralanguage includes pauses and hesitation; accent; sighing, screaming, laughing, crying and whistling; and 'guggles', for example 'Uh huh and 'M mm'

Verbal communication

In general NVC is more important for interpersonal relations whilst verbal communication is more important for exchanging information and practical tasks. According to Trower et al (1978) there are eight different kinds of verbal communication or utterances, with quite different functions.

These are:
1. Instructions and directions
2. Questions
3. Comments, suggestions and information
4. Informal chat or gossip
5. Performative utterances
6. Social routines
7. Expressive emotions or attitudes
8. Latent messages.

1. Instructions and directions

These are intended to directly affect the behaviour of another person and vary from mild suggestions to commands.

2. Questions

These are intended to influence the verbal behaviour of others by requesting information, whether factual or otherwise and thus eliciting a reply. Questions have many functions, for example, to arouse interest or curiosity by focussing attention on a particular issue, or to initiate an encounter or to show concern or caring towards another.

Hargie et al (1981) describes seven different types of questions. These are: recall and process, closed and open, affective; leading, rhetorical, multiple and probing. The type used will depend upon the social context and the response required. For example some types will be more suitable when interviewing a patient, whilst others are more suitable when teaching.

3. Comments, suggestions and information

These are given in direct response to questions or as independent comments or suggestions on other people's utterances. Factual information may be imported in relation to the carrying out of practical tasks or during a lecture.

4. Informal chat or gossip

A great deal of social behaviour consists of 'small talk' where behaviour is largely unaffected and little important information is exchanged, such as in the telling of jokes. The function of chat or gossip is mainly for mutual enjoyment and usually occurs in more informal social situations, such as at a party.

5. Performative utterances

These have immediate social consequences which constitute their meaning and are usually uttered at specific social events. They include opening fetes, launching ships, christening babies, passing verdicts and apologising or making promises.

6. Social routines

These are culturally-bound social routines which may be classified into five main kinds. Routines for greetings and partings; for initiating and changing situations; for confirming, supporting and giving; for remedies (apologies and accounts); and routines for asserting rights and refusing. Most people are aware of these routines, but failure to use them correctly may offend or even insult and may result in possible rejection of the individual.

7. Expressing emotions or attitudes

These are more often and more accurately expressed non-verbally, but verbal expressions may serve to emphasise the non-verbal expression of emotions or attitudes. For example, 'I am feeling very depressed', or 'I like you'. Negative feelings, however, towards people, are more often verbalised if the person concerned is not present, for example, 'She makes me really angry'.

8. Latent messages

These may be intentional or unintentional and include the same sort of questions or information as in the other examples. However, these may be expressed in a number of different ways to imply a different or further meaning. For instance, 'Have you stopped beating your wife yet?' is a well known example of a latent message.

Social skills model

So far we have looked at some definitions of social skills and described the main elements of non-verbal and verbal communication. Now we need to look at a model of social skills which draws these elements together and emphasises the importance of feedback in the motivation to achieve social goals. It also indicates ways in which social performances can fail and how training procedures may effectively improve—through an analogy with motor skills training (Argyle & Kendon, 1967).

Argyle explains that 'this model conceptualises man as pursuing social and other goals, acting according to rules and monitoring his performance in the light of continuous feedback from the environment'.

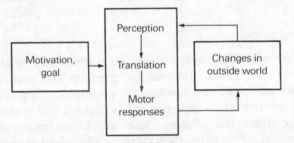

Fig. 7.1 The social skills model (Argyle, 1967).

Motivation and goals

Goals may be general or specific. If we take the analogy between motor skills and social skills, then the motor skill operator may have the general goal of becoming an excellent tennis player and the specific goal of speeding up his serve. In social skills, a general goal may be to learn to be at ease at a party, whilst a specific goal might be to learn how to initiate a conversation with a stranger. Goals may also be either long or short-term. A long-term motor-skill goal might be to win Wimbledon some day and a short-term one to win to-day's club match. Similarly, a long-term social skill might be to become a TV interviewer, a short-term (or sub-goal) might be to learn how to ask interesting questions.

Goals may be very definite, for example, a door-to-door salesman wanting to change attitudes or beliefs. Goals may be motivated simply by basic social needs such as biological needs, dependency, affiliation, dominance, sex, aggression and self-esteem. These innate needs may stimulate unconscious motivation, whilst the more definite goals are more consciously motivated. Usually, there is a mixture of both conscious and unconscious motivations. For example, the salesman may also unconsciously want to dominate the customer or impress his boss.

Translation

This applies to the process whereby the individual translates the perceptions he receives into a plan of action. Initially, this process may take place at a conscious level, but as the person gains experience it becomes sub-conscious or automatic. Thus, a car driver will decide he should start to slow down and stop when he perceives the lights changing. This decision is chosen from a range of behaviours as being the most suitable for the circumstances (and from his knowledge of the Highway Code). As he gains experience, this translation will become automatic. Similarly, if a girl goes to a party on her own, and a smiling, well-dressed man comes up and asks her to dance, she must translate all these perceptions in order to respond.

Response

At this point the skill becomes manifest in terms of a responsive behaviour—whether non-verbal or vocal or verbal. The car driver applies his brakes to slow down and stop at the lights. The party goer either smiles back, replies or else avoids all contact and moves away. The individual's response system has turned the plan or translation into observable behaviour or response.

Feedback—changes in outside world

Feedback from the environment is occurring all the time through non-verbal and vocal and verbal clues. This allows the individual to assess the effects of his behaviour and to modify his subsequent behaviour in the light of it.

The car driver may have braked too sharply and the car behind nearly run into him (so the next time he approaches changing traffic lights, he will glance in his rear view mirror before applying his brakes). The party-goer finds that when she gives a friendly response, she is drawn into an interesting conversation and begins to feel more at ease. (In future she may feel less apprehensive about going to a party unattached.)

Perception

We are gaining information and feedback from our environment all the time. These come through our main sensory channels—sight, sound, smell, taste and touch. Sight and sound are the most important in social interaction. Furthermore, perception is an active rather than a passive process. Thus, it is possible to train a person to pick up relevant clues in interpersonal communication, such as watching facial expression or hearing the tone of voice or listening to what is actually said.

This social skills model by Argyle provides a framework by which we can identify each step or action or component of social interaction. It also allows us to analyse where a person may be more competent or less competent.

Social competence

A mistake often made is of thinking that a person who is 'socially competent' is so in every given situation. There is no evidence to show that such a paragon exists. Rather, we are all more skilled in some situations than in others. For example, the brilliant speaker may baulk at asking a girl out; the perfect hostess may be nervous at a committee meeting.

Another common mistake is to think that a social skill is always used for a social purpose. The gifted speaker may entertain his audience, the relaxed hostess will make her guests feel welcome and at ease. However, these results may not always be advantages to the recipient. In both cases, the social skills may be employed for an anti-social purpose. His ulterior motive may be to sell his latest book, her's to sell her newest line in cosmetics.

Social competence, or the individual's ability to produce the desired effect on, or response from, other people, is more easily defined in the case of professional social skills. For example, a competent or skilled ballet dancer receives more curtain calls; a competent or skilled doctor cures more patients. But it is much less easy to define success is relation to everyday social skills, such as talking to the neighbours or coping with aggression. Conversely, lack of social competence is relatively easier to identify, especially when it is marked.

Social inadequacy

What is meant by this lack of competence or social inadequacy and what are its causes? What are the characteristics of a socially inadequate person?

Nature

First of all, social inadequacy may be measured in behavioural terms. And as we have already outlined, behavioural and learning theories suggest that social skills are acquired from childhood. Learning occurs through experience, both seeing and doing, that is, partly through observation and imitation of others, partly through negative and positive reinforcement and extrinsic and intrinsic reinforcement, partly through cognitive development and partly through innate potential. Humanistic theories suggest that the development of social skills is part of an individual's conscious and unconscious drive towards self-actualisation.

Cause

Social inadequacy may come about through a number of complex reasons. But in general, research shows that a person lacking in social skills is one who has been deprived of adequate models of social behaviour in his parents, siblings, peers or other significant figures of influence. There may also be genetic influences in that the innate predispositions of the child actively influence his social experiences. Thus both innate and environmental influences play their part in helping or preventing the individual from learning or practising an adequate range of social behaviours.

Characteristics

A socially inadequate person may be defined as being unable to produce the desired effect on the behaviour and feelings of other people that he wants and which society accepts. Such a person will appear isolated, cold, inept, unassertive, bad-tempered and generally unrewarding. He has difficulty in communicating with others and in forming and sustaining meaningful relationships.

Links with mental health

It must be stating the obvious to say that there are strong links between social inadequacy and mental health; from the person who experiences unease when engaged in conversation, to the with-drawal of the chronic schizophrenic patient. Many people suffer as a result of being socially unskilled and in a wide variety of social situations. However, the cut-off point between what is 'normal' and what becomes a social behaviour problem, is essentially when the person asks for, or agrees to accept help. The distinction lies in the degree to which the problem disrupts their lives.

From studies of the 'normal' population it has been found that at least 7 per cent suffer from serious difficulties with social behaviour. Studies of psychiatric patients indicate an even greater proportion. It has also been found that social inadequacy may occur in one of two main patterns—either as a primary or as a secondary factor.

Primary

Social inadequacy may be primary, leading to rejection and further social isolation and in turn, producing disturbed mental states. For example, the young girl who has been brought up alone by an over-anxious mother, is sent to an all-girls' school, has few girlfriends and no boyfriends, feels rejected, becomes isolated and develops a clinical depression.

Secondary

Other kinds of mental disorders affect all areas of behaviour including social behaviour, which, in turn, lead to rejection and social isolation and so add to the initial source of distress. For example, the above process may work in reverse with the clinical depression leading to rejection, isolation and socially inadequate behaviour.

It is also worth noting that the concept of social inadequacy implies some element of persisting behaviour. It is less concerned with the transient disruption of social skills, due to the onset of the psychiatric illness and more to do with the probable preceding history of social difficulties.

Selection of patients for SST

Selection of patients for training in social skills is based on the ex-tent of their social inadequacy or 'the degree of subjective dissatis-faction with the performance of adult social roles, that leads to an avoidance of those situations where an appropriate performance of these roles is obligation' (Falloon et al 1974).

It is, of course, most important that this selection be carried out on an individual basis, as each patient will have their own specific needs in given situations. However, although there is a danger of using diagnostic labels and losing sight of the individual, it is possible and perhaps helpful for selection purposes, to slot some forms of social inadequacy into general diagnostic categories.

Depressive states

Patients with depressive illnesses also tend to have a low level of motor and verbal activity. Movements are retarded and the posture drooped or tense. Speech is also often slow, low in tone and expressionless. There may be little eye contact as the gaze is downcast and the facial expression is often sad and gloomy. The person appears tired, apathetic and lacking in initiative, and often suffers from feelings of guilt, and unworthiness and anxiety. Social contact will be avoided due to loss of interest in other people. These poor social skills and unrewarding behaviour mean that there is little reinforcement from others, which in turn, leads to the depressed condition.

Anxiety states

In the case of patients suffering from anxiety states, the prolonged and anxious feelings result in increase of motor and verbal activity. Movements may be sharp and uncontrolled and posture tense. Speech is often breathless and comes in short rapid bursts. Eye contact is fleeting and the expression preoccupied and worried. The anxiety is often further increased through over-sensitivity to others and self-consciousness in social situations. The anxious person may transmit his disquiet to others so strongly that he is avoided and this in turn adds to his anxiety.

Phobic states

A similar picture is seen in the case of patients suffering from social phobias. Here, the person experiences exaggerated and irrational fear in such situations as parties, interviews or dates with the opposite sex. Claustrophobia (fear of enclosed spaces) and agroraphobia (fear of open spaces) are two other main phobias which affect the person's social adequacy, and which may lead to further isolation and increased anxiety.

Obsessive compulsive states

Social anxiety and inadequacy may also be experienced by those
suffering from obsessive/compulsive states. Such patients become
continually and morbidly preoccupied with certain ideas or actions
and may as a result withdraw socially and become isolated.

Alcoholism and drug addiction

Alcoholics and drug addicts are also found to be deficient in certain
social skills, especially the skills required to cope with the stresses
of life (other than resorting to drink or drugs) and the skills needed
to resist social pressures to keep on taking them. In addition to
assertiveness, these patients require skills to make them feel less
inferior and more acceptable to others.

Behavioural problems and personality disorders

Children and adolescents showing either withdrawn, unassertive
behaviour or aggressive, disturbed behaviour, tend to be unpopu-
lar. This unpopularity is associated with poor social skills. Social
inadequacy may in turn lead to delinquency, imprisonment and/or
mental illness, which may include psychopathic and abnormal
personality disorders. In all these cases many social skills may need
to be re-learned or learned, particularly assertive skills with less
aggression and skills to increase self-worth by eliciting more positive responses from the other person.

Epilepsy

Patients suffering from convulsions, seizures or fits may often be
frightened by their epilepsy and other people's reactions to it and
them. Thus, they may react by adopting aggressive behaviour or
by withdrawing from social situations. Either way their behaviour
may be socially inadequate and may lead to isolation and
depression.

Schizophrenia

Patients with schizophrenia (especially those suffering from chronic
schizophrenia), often present with the most extreme forms of social
inadequacy. These include withdrawal, lack of spontaneous and

relevant verbal communication and flattening of emotion. Non-verbal communication is also lacking, particularly eye contact, body posture, gesture and facial expression. There is often a failure on the part of the patient to make or maintain close relationships. (In long-term psychiatry there is a failure to cope with everyday personal-care skills, such as washing and dressing; or simple literacy and numeracy skills such as reading, writing, telling the time and counting money.)

Having looked at these main diagnostic categories to discover some common forms of social inadequacies it must be remembered that within each, there is a wide range of differences between individuals. However, they give us some indication of the sort of problems which the patient may suffer from and which may be helped through training in social skills.

Individual assessment

Further assessment of each individual patient should be made to discover more about their past and present relationships and what kind of enduring problems they have with various people; also to find out more about difficulties they experience in specific situations and the particular inadequate behaviours which they show in these situations.

Information should be obtained from other staff or relatives, from interviews with the patient, or from observing the patient's interaction with others. Records and ratings may also be made from these observations and when all the relevant information is gathered together, a suitable SST programme can be planned to meet the patient's individual needs.

The SST programme may be tailor-made to carry out with the patient on his own, or he may join a group of patients with similar problems. This standard training is in the form of a set course, covering all the important basic social skills in a systematic way. This set programme may also be carried out on an individual basis but there are obvious social advantages of working in a closed group and in the majority of cases is the preferred approach.

SOCIAL SKILLS TRAINING

Training in social skills has developed rapidly in the past few years and has learned much from alternative approaches to skills training such as: 'interaction' and 'transactional' analysis; 'encounter', 'sensitivity' and 'T' groups; 'psychodrama' and 'assertiveness' training. However, SST should not be confused with these other approaches, because, although they may have similar objectives, the methods used in some cases are entirely different.

Even within the SST approach, there may be variations in the training programme due to such factors as the number and needs of patients, number and experience of staff and the time, space and equipment available. Various SST programmes are described lescents (Hanlon, 1977); with prisoners (Fawcett et al, 1979); with alcoholics and drug addicts (Van Hassett, 1978); with epileptics (Westland, 1980) and with chronic psychiatric patients (Robertson, 1978).

Example of SST programme

Yet another approach—which will be described here in more detail, as it is suitable for use in acute psychiatry with a variety of patient groups—is by Falloon et al (1974). This is outlined in a 'Social Training' Manual, which describes training methods in social behaviour at the Psychological Training Centre, Maudsley Hospital, London. The subjects include those with specific social phobias, depression, schizophrenia, obsessional states, sexual disorders and dependency on alcohol and drugs.

The SST course lasts ten weeks with one 75 minute session per week (first 10 minutes, discussion of 'homework'; 60 minutes, demonstration and practise of difficult social situations; last 5 minutes, setting goals for next week.)

It is designed specifically to improve the competency of 'socially inadequate' subjects (as defined). The training takes place in small groups with six to eight subjects and male and female co-leaders. Techniques used include modelling, role play, didactic teaching material (handouts), group discussion and activity, and an operant home programme.

Training is divided into ten hierarchical stages, including the basic non-verbal and verbal communication skills already described in this chapter. A week before each session the subject is given a handout with the principles outlined and any questions may be discussed at the start of the session. Relaxation techniques are taught as an appropriate method of coping with anxiety (rather than using alcohol or drugs).

Group discussion, modelling, role play and practice take place at each session. Goals for the incoming week are set at the end of each session and each subject keeps a diary of ten target behaviours to be practised in real life situations (operant home programme). Much positive feedback is given in the group, but it is essential that the subject learns to provide his own self-reinforcement. (Partial success is regarded as nearing complete success, rather than just another failure.)

This model is SST, based on Argyle's approach to social skills learning, provides the person with an opportunity to learn new social skills and roles or to improve existing ones. It also encourages transfer of learning from the workshop to the real-life situation.

The ten stages of training sessions are in brief:

(Please see Falloon et al (1974) for details.)

1. *Non-verbal communication*

   Discussion—introduction, posture, anxiety, relaxation, group norms.

   Practice—relaxation techniques, coping self-talk.

2. *Non-verbal expression*

   Discussion—gaze, touch, appearance.

   Practice—shaking hands with eye contact

3. *Vocal expression*

   Discussion—importance of voice control and style in different situations.

   Practice—different types of conversation in pairs using different tones and styles.

4. *Simple verbal expression*

   Discussion—importance of appropriate links with NVC.

   Practice—greetings, introductions, expanding on yes/no answers.

5. *Work situations*

   Discussion—job selection and interviews.

   Practice—interviews, being interviewer and interviewee, asking for a rise.

6. *Expressing feelings*

   Discussion—importance of expressing feelings at the time.

   Practice—expressing anger, affection, approval, disapproval, love.

7. *Group interaction*

   Discussion—different groups, family, work, social. Feeling in or out of groups.

   Practice—any group discussion.

8. *Initiating friendships*

Discussion—need of friends, how to meet people.

Practice—starting conversations with same or opposite sex.

9. *Sexual behaviour*

Discussion—initiating contact, kissing, cuddling and anxieties about specific behaviour.

Practice—difficulties are obvious, but good quality audio-visual material could be used to promote discussion.

10. *Revision*

Discussion or practice in any or all of the above as required.

Assessment is carried out the week before and the week after the course and again three, six and nine months after completion. Change is measured largely on self-assessment and progress made on the ten target problems in real-life situations. A standardised interview is used in assessment, plus a videotaped behavioural test of non-verbal and verbal performance.

On completion of the course each person is encouraged to use the SST framework taught in his everyday life; to continue to set up new short-term goals; to use self-reinforcement for competent performance and to work step by step towards the long term goal of obtaining satisfaction and enjoyment from his social activities and relationships.

Occupational therapy and SST

It is perhaps not surprising that the recent interest in training in social skills has been taken up by many of the paramedical professions, including occupational therapists (some studies have already been quoted). The occupational therapy and SST approach to rehabilitation has much in common. The symbol of the mythical phoenix bird adopted by our profession, represents the individual's part in his own 'renewal'. It is with the help of the therapist and through the patient's own efforts that he is motivated and able to change. This self-help notion is also central to SST.

The occupational therapist views her patient as a whole person and this inevitably means assessment of his social abilities and inadequacies in his own unique social situation. Social inadequacy causes suffering. It is the job of the therapist to help return the patient to his fullest possible social competence. And one method is through the use of SST programmes.

Training in social skills may be seen to have a number of advantages and disadvantages. A resumé of the main ones may help to define the scope and possible limitations of SST as an approach to treatment in acute psychiatry.

Advantages of SST

1. It has a theoretical base, but is behaviour orientated and therefore more practical and transferable from workshop to real-life situations.
2. It allows an individual's social behaviour and specific skills to be analysed in set situations.
3. It allows the examination of appropriate social roles and feelings about own and other's roles.
4. It encourages re-learning of old social skills and learning of new more appropriate ones.
5. It is suitable for a wide variety of patient groups, including both in- and out-patients, male and female, young and old.
6. It may take place in small groups rather than on a one-to-one basis, which has both practical and social advantages.
7. Results may be seen relatively quickly in comparison with other more long-term forms of treatment.
8. It is adaptable to the needs of specific patients.
9. It is a 'positive' form of treatment as it depends more on the learning of skills than on having a particular type of personality.
10. It encourages self-esteem and feelings of self-worth and helps to lower anxiety levels in particular social situations.
11. It allows the individual to have more control of his own behaviour and environment.
12. It is relatively easy to set up in terms of space and (simple) equipment.

Disadvantages of SST

1. May be expensive to set up if videotape-recorders or one-way viewing mirrors are used.
2. May require therapists to have special training
3. The response of the individual to standard programmes may differ greatly and some may find the approach too threatening.
4. Improvements may be difficult to maintain on a long term basis.
5. Transference of learning from the workshop to real-life situations may be difficult if these are limited.

Summary

From a variety of studies (some mentioned), it has been found that social skills training in acute psychiatry has more advantages than disadvantages and that patients certainly benefit at least in the short term.

However, the model of treatment adopted depends not only on the occupational therapist, but also on the whole ethos of the hospital or unit within which she works as a member of an integrated team. If she wishes to implement a SST programme she must first gain knowledge of a theoretical and practical nature in order to argue a stronger case (various SST courses are now available for professional staff). The therapist herself requires to be suitably skilled in a range of basic social behaviours, as inevitably, the patients will follow her example.

It is also preferable that she shares the organisation and running of such training programmes with a similarly qualified co-leader and preferably one of the opposite sex, as mixed sex groups require both female and male models. Equipment may be kept to a minimum. Videotape-recorders and one-way mirrors are useful, but not essential—as patients' behaviour may be 'played back' through role-play.

She also needs a quiet room with easy chairs and an uninterrupted weekly or bi-weekly slot in the timetable. Lastly, but most importantly, she needs to select a 'suitable' patient group.

Apart from all the practical aspects, she also needs to have enthusiasm for the task and sensitive awareness of her patients' needs. Communication is a two-way process, but the main responsibility will lie with the occupational therapist. Social skills training is not an end in itself, but a means to an end. That is to help the patient to reach his fullest possible social competence and to lead as enjoyable and satisfying a life as possible within his community.

REFERENCES

Argyle M (ed) 1981 Social skills and health. Methuen, London
Argyle M 1978 The psychology of interpersonal behaviour. Penguin, Harmondsworth
Argyle M, Kendon A 1967 The experimental analysis of social performance. In Berkowitz L (ed) Advances in experimental social psychology 3: 55–58. Academic Press, New York
Bandura A L 1971 Social learning theory. General Learning Press, New York
Birdwhistell R L 1970 Kinesics and context. University of Pennsylvania Press, Philadelphia
Bowlby J 1969 Attachment. Basic Books, New York

Combs M L, Slazby D A 1977 Social skills training with children. In: Lahey
    B B, Kazin A E (eds) Advances in clinical child psychology. Plenum Press,
    New York
Falloon I, Lindley P, McDonald R 1974 Social training—a manual. Psychological
    Treatment Section, Maudsley Hospital London SE5
Fawcett B, Ingham E, McKeever M, Williams S 1979 Social skills group for
    young prisoners. Social Work To-day 10: 16–18
Friedman N, Hoffman S P 1967 Kinetic behaviour in altered clinical states.
    Perceptual and Motor Skills 24: 525–39
Froebal F 1887 The education of man. Kelley, New Jersey
Hall E T 1959 The silent language. Doubleday, New York
Hanlon S 1977 Social skills training with disturbed adolescents. British Journal of
    Occupational Therapy 40: 271–272
Hargie O, Saunders C, Dickson D 1981 Social skills in interpersonal
    communication. Croom Helm, London
Harlow H F, Harlow M K 1966 Learning to love. American Scientist, 54: 244–72
Jourard S 1966 An exploratory study of body accessability. British Journal of
    Social and Clinical Psychology 5: 221–31
Maslow A H 1954 Motivation and personality. Harper and Row, New York
Osgood C E 1966 Dimensionality of the semantic space for communication via
    facial expression. Scandinavian Journal of Psychology 7: 1–30
Robertson J M 1978 Ideas for materials and social skills assessment. British
    Journal of Occupational Therapy 41: 365–367
Rogers C 1965 Client centred therapy. Constable, London
Rutter M 1972 Material deprivation reassessed. Penguin, Harmondsworth
The Concise Oxford Dictionary 1980 University Press, Oxford
Trower P, Bryant B, Argyle M 1978 Social skills and mental health. Methuen,
    London
Van Haselt V, Hersen M, Milliones J 1978 Social skills training for alcoholics and
    drug addicts — a review. Addictive Behaviours 3: 221–233
Westland G 1980 Social skills training with epileptic psychiatric patients. British
    Journal of Occupational Therapy 43: 13–16

RECOMMENDED READING

Argyle M 1975 Bodily communication. Methuen, London
Argyle M 1973 Social interaction. Aldine Pub. Co., Chicago
Argyle M (ed) 1981 Social skills and health. Methuen, London
Argyle M 1978 The psychology of Interpersonal behaviour. Penguin,
    Harmondsworth
Avila D, Combs A W, Purkey W (eds) 1977 The helping relationship source
    book. Allyn and Bacon Inc, Boston
Becvar R J 1974 Skills for effective communication: a guide to building
    relationships. John Wiley & Sons, New York
Bellack A S, Hersen M 1979 Research and practice in social skills training.
    Plenum Press, New York and London
Berne E 1967 Games people play. Grove Press, New York
Douglas T 1979 Groupwork practice. Tavistock Publications, London
Eisler R M, Frederikson L W 1980 Perfecting social skills. Plenum Press, New
    York and London
Ellis R, Whittington D 1981 A guide to social skill training. Croom Helm,
    London
Falloon I, Lindley P, McDonald R 1974 Social training — a manual.
    Psychological Treatment Section, Maudsley Hospital, London SE5

Hilgard E R, Atkinson C A, Atkinson R L 1975 Introduction to psychology. Harcourt Brace Jovanovich Inc., New York

Priestley P, McGuire J, Flegg D, Hemsley V, Welham D 1978 Social skills and personal problem solving — a handbook of methods. Tavistock Pub., London.

Remocker A J Storch E T 1982 Action speaks louder, 3rd edn. Churchill Livingstone, Edinburgh

Rogers C 1967 Client centred therapy. Constable, London

Smith D R, Williamson L K 1979 Interpersonal communication. William Brown Co., Iowa

Sprott W J H 1975 Human groups. Penguin , Harmondsworth

Trower P, Bryant B, Argyle M 1978 Social skills and mental health. Methuen, London

Willson M 1983 Occupational therapy in long term psychiatry. Churchill Livingstone, Edinburgh

The management of anxiety

MANIFESTATIONS OR ANXIETY

Normal anxiety

Anxiety and the autonomic nervous system

The autonomic nervous system keeps the body functioning by allowing the heart to beat and respiration to continue without conscious control. This system can be divided into the sympathetic and the parasympathetic branches. The sympathetic branch is the energy utilising division which speeds up the rate at which the body works. The parasympathetic branch conserves energy and is used during sleep and digestion for example.

The effects and symptoms of arousal

The human body has evolved over millions of years yet still retains within the nervous system some of the basic responses which would have been useful to our early ancestors. The caveman suddenly faced with a charging mammoth had to make an instantaneous decision—fight or flight.

Whichever he chose, the autonomic nervous system allowed for maximum efficiency. Within the body adrenalin was released into the bloodstream to increase the heart-rate which in turn improved the blood flow. At the same time respiration would increase allowing more oxygen into the circulatory system which directed an improved blood supply to the voluntary muscles which were tensed for action.

This increased activity by the somatic systems produced heat and water as by-products which were lost through the skin by flushing and perspiration. The improved blood supply to the voluntary muscles caused a sinking, nauseous feeling in the stomach and often

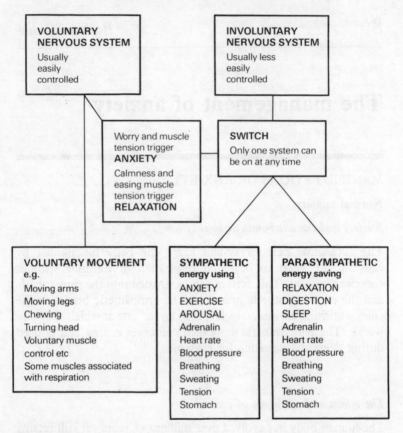

Fig. 8.1 The nervous system: a simplified model (Miller, 1979).

the bladder and bowel would be evacuated to reduce the body weight before activity.

This response to stress is useful today when an individual meets a challenge. From time to time the media reports superhuman feats performed under stress. For example, a mother may have bodily lifted the rear wheel of a car to allow rescuers to remove her injured child, trapped under the rear wheel; impossible under normal circumstances.

Likewise, the challenge of performing well on stage or during an examination is met by this response which allows for an improved performance.

Anxiety is a biological defence mechanism which warns of potential danger and leads to some form of response in order to deal with the situation.

Neurotic anxiety

Inappropriate responses

When the defence mechanism of flight or fight is activated in response to an anxiety-provoking situation and the response is disproportionate to the stimulus the arising symptoms cause it to be termed 'neurotic anxiety'.

Although anxiety may be appropriate when the body is endangered it is inappropriate in potentially 'safe' situations such as when standing in a bar with friends.

Clinical conditions

Neurotic anxiety presents in many forms and is a major component in a wide range of clinical conditions:

Phobic states: agoraphobia; social phobia; illness phobia; animal phobia; claustrophobia etc.

Anxiety states: anticipatory anxiety; free-floating anxiety; obsessional anxiety; neurotic depression; examination anxiety etc.

Stress problems: insomnia; overwork, writer's cramp; stammering; loss of concentration and memory; irritability; marital stress; difficulty in decision making; hysterical disorders etc.

Psychosomatic problems: duodenal ulcers; angina of effort; asthma; migraine; tension headaches; hypertension; chronic indigestion; somatic aches and pains etc.

Sexual dysfunction: secondary impotence; vaginismus; premature ejaculation; dyspareunia; orgasmic dysfunction etc.

Rehabilitation problems: following C.V.A., myocardial infarction; physical handicap; plastic surgery etc.

Neurotic anxiety saps the individual's energy, initiative and interest in life and leaves the therapist with the initial problem of remotivating the clients sufficiently to ensure their active participation in their treatment programme.

Manifestation of symptoms

The neurotic client faced with a mild stimulus feels palpitations as the heart rate increases and muscles become tense. The tension in the muscles of the chest wall and throat causes a feeling of tightness or choking and the client hyperventilates in an attempt to improve the air supply to the lungs. The face becomes flushed and the skin perspires as the body tries to lose heat. Dizziness, tingling of the peripheries and pounding or ringing in the ears may occur due to the increased blood pressure.

As tension increases within the muscles they begin to tighten and tremble. Stammering may occur when the muscles associated with speech are affected and nausea or fluttering when the stomach muscles contract quickly.

Awareness of these symptoms aggravates the situation. The feeling that there is something wrong with the client's bodily functions increases tension which further exacerbates the symptoms. The result is an anxiety spiral which culminates in panic and a desire to run away.

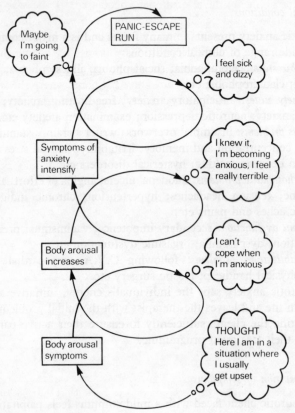

Fig. 8.2 The anxiety spiral.

The phobic client

Neurotic anxiety frequently develops into a phobic state, the most commonly treated being agoraphobia and social phobia.

The classical history given by an agoraphobic client is that whilst queueing in a supermarket, she became aware of the symptoms of increased tension. She may have been unwell that day or been late for an important appointment, aggravated by the need to queue.

As tension increased, she felt palpitation as her heart rate increased and a constriction of her throat. As she hyperventilated in an effort to increase her air supply she became faint and a cold sweat broke out making her feel nauseous. She was afraid that she would collapse and draw attention to herself which further increased the level of tension until the panic state of flight was reached. She quickly left the supermarket and hurried home.

In her home the level of anxiety decreased. If she was sick or fainted there would be no embarrassment. She was safe.

The fear that the same symptoms may have arisen again had caused her to become reluctant to leave home. Each time she tried she became anxious, observed the symptoms and did not know how to cope with them. She therefore stayed at home where she was safe and her behaviour was reinforced. A vicious circle had been allowed to develop and intervention was necessary if her behaviour was to change.

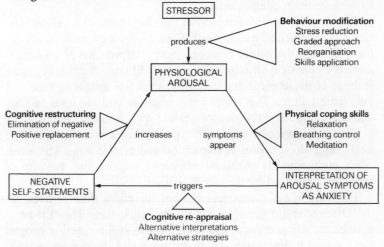

Fig. 8.3 Intervention in anxiety management—an extension of the model proposed by Jaremko (1979).

Stress related disease

Neurotic anxiety plays a major role in the development of many physical illnesses. Clients presenting with angina pectoris, hypertension or rheumatoid disease are often found to be very precise, demanding people who set and attain very high standards for themselves. They often refuse to accept that they are anxious or stressed but will admit that they are perfectionists. To admit that they are stressed is seen as a weakness and falls below their high standards. They may not feel that they need to learn the skill of relaxation and may not feel able to delegate tasks to others whilst they attend a relaxation course because they like to be in control of all events in their lives.

The overworked businessman is a candidate for heart disease at an early age because of the nature of his lifestyle. Long hours of work, lack of regular exercise, rushed meals and stress addition are factors leading to this. For this reason many international corporations send their executives on Anxiety Management Courses in an effort to reduce the number of days lost by valued members of staff becoming ill.

Anxiety states

Miller, Cullen and O'Brien (1981) reported that 'Anxiety states have three main components:

The *cognitive* component is what the client thinks or feels in relation to the experience of anxiety. Commonly, a client is poorly informed about the nature of anxiety and interprets his physiological arousal as physical or mental illness. In addition clients may report feelings of detachment and unreality; they feel unable to cope and anticipate failure. This increasingly negative attitude leads to poor and inappropriate strategies for dealing with stressful situations.

The *physiological* component typically consists of increases in heart rate, blood pressure, respiration and muscle tone. These and other autonomically mediated responses underly the majority of symptoms reported by the anxious client.

The *behavioural* component is what the client does or does not do. Often stressful situations are avoided altogether. Thus the agoraphobic avoids going out, the social phobic avoids meeting people, the stressed businessman avoids decisions and the person recovering from a heart attack may avoid any exercise.

Such avoidance can have disastrous and occasionally lethal consequences. The client may become unable to lead a normal useful life. Even when situations are faced we may find that the client's repertoire of behaviour is inadequate, inappropriate or severely disrupted by stress and arousal.'

THE REDUCTION OF ANXIETY

Overcoming anxiety

Drugs and alcohol

Anxiety is easily reduced by the administration of alcohol. This depressant of the central nervous system is readily available and socially acceptable. Many busy people like to unwind with a drink after a hard day.

Unfortunately, if alcohol is relied upon regularly to reduce anxiety it loses its effect. One drink no longer depresses the central nervous system and the drinker resorts to taking larger amounts of alcohol to obtain the desired feelings of relaxation. A physiological and psychological dependence arises with the drinker often requiring treatment for alcoholism which may further add to the anxiety state.

Drugs too are easily available. Many stressful people cannot cope with their lives because of unemployment, poor housing, lack of money, loneliness or inharmonious interpersonal relationships. They present to overworked General Practitioners with the symptoms of anxiety and are prescribed tranquillisers. The drugs relieve their symptoms by deadening their ability to perceive their environment which is the anxiety-producing stimulus. The effect of the drugs is short-lived and the need occurs to increase the dose in order that the original effect is achieved, often resulting in a drug dependent state.

Treating anxiety with tranquillisers is an expensive use of national resources. It is estimated that twenty to thirty million prescriptions are issued for these drugs each year in Great Britain.

Yoga

Yoga is a popular form of exercise which produces a feeling of relaxation and well-being. It is a method of development for body and mind originating from the Far East and is intended as a complete system of self-improvement. Many clients may benefit from this system which requires exercises to be practised daily in a quiet location.

For some clients, the Yogis (people who practise Yoga) have become confused with the Fakirs from India who have gained extraordinary control of their senses in order to subject their bodies to abnormal conditions such as lying on beds of nails. The client may feel uncomfortable with this association of ideas and be unable to accept the beliefs of Yoga which link it with Mysticism.

In addition, clients who have not exercised regularly and are past their youth may find great difficulty in carrying out the required movements, although Yogis insist that the exercises can be performed with ease by people 'from four to forty' (Hittleman, 1971).

For those clients who are able to enjoy Yoga it is an excellent method of gaining control of body and mind.

Cognitive Behaviour Modification

Cognitive Behaviour Modification became popular in the 1970s as a treatment for anxiety based problems and is widely used today. It uses the techniques of relaxation, systematic desensitisation, graded practice and cognitive re-orientation and is a cost effective method of treatment. Because clients may be treated in groups, the number of staff hours per patient required may be reduced and the development of self-help groups is possible.

There are no adverse side-effects nor tolerance problems and the techniques are invaluable in Health Education and Primary Care. The keystones of this form of treatment are education, skills acquisition and their application.

Cognitive Behaviour Modification has currently developed into Anxiety Management Training which teaches the client to 'manage' anxiety which is a natural response and cannot be 'cured'.

Anxiety Management Training

Strategies

Anxiety Management Training aims to treat the three main components of anxiety states; the cognitive, the physiological and the behavioural components. It allows for:

1. *The provision of accurate information about the nature of anxiety.* It provides information which stresses that anxiety is a natural state which the client must learn to control and teaches the skills with which to do it. As with any other skill it may be broken down into simple components which may be easily learned and will provide for the life-long management of anxiety.

2. *The recognition of negative attitudes.* Clients who are anxious tend to make negative self-statements which increases anxiety, and

the therapist will demonstrate this. A simple method is to suggest to the group that each member will be required to give a short talk on a topic of their choice later in the session. Generally, they will respond by thinking 'I can't do that. I am going to make a fool of myself' etc. accompanied by feelings of anxiety arousal and a desire to escape.

Ten or fifteen minutes later, the therapist will reassure the group members that they do not have to make a speech after all and will ask each of them to describe their earlier feelings. Usually, the pattern of negative self-statements and the physiological arousal will have given way at a point where a positive, coping self-statement has been made, for example, 'Well I could talk about that play I saw on T.V. last night' or 'No one will expect too much of me'. These positive cognitions will have produced a reduction in anxiety levels and the exercise will have demonstrated to the clients the effectiveness of both negative and positive self-statements.

3. *The acquisition of positive attitudes and coping cognitive strategies.* Clients generally develop a habit of anticipating anxiety in that they prepare to meet a difficult situation by worrying about the things that might go wrong. Positive planning, involving a realistic assessment of the likely difficulties combined with the consideration of alternative coping strategies, must replace anticipation anxiety. Clients must be encouraged to concentrate on ways to succeed rather than on ways to fail.

4. *The recognition of the onset of physiological symptoms.* Clients may be taught to monitor the gross changes in their physiological state. They can learn that the observance of an increased pulse rate and the presence of muscular tension during a stressful situation will signify the need to put into practice the relaxation techniques until the stress is reduced to an acceptable level, before proceeding with the activity.

In the initial stages of training, it is useful if bio-feedback equipment is available to demonstrate the changes occurring during tense and relaxed states. The most commonly used equipment is the Galvanic Skin Response monitor (G.S.R.) which measures the increased wetness of the skin when the client is subjected to stress. The electrode pads are fastened to the client's fingertips and he is able to observe the changing levels on a monitor. It is usually possible to have an audible tone which rises in pitch with increased anxiety and falls during relaxation.

For a more sophisticated approach, the G.S.R. may be linked to a computer which will flash information onto its visual display unit.

The messages are directly related to the client's level of arousal or relaxation e.g. 'Well done. You are relaxing well' or 'your anxiety level is increasing. Try and relax a little more'.

Changes can be produced experimentally by a number of simple procedures ranging from imagining a distressing situation to production of the 'startle response' to a loud noise. If a warning is given before the noise is produced anticipation anxiety may be demonstrated.

5. *The acquisition of relaxation skills and self-control*. Relaxation training can take a number of forms. Techniques of even, regular breathing are the simplest, though methods such as listening to a metronome or bio-feedback training have been successfully employed.

The most commonly used technique is that which developed from the work of Jacobson (1938) on progressive muscular relaxation. Clients using this method are taught to distinguish between tension and relaxation within different muscle groups and learn to achieve deep levels of relaxation, and it is this technique which forms the basis for the more recently developed 'Anxiety Management Programme'.

6. *The application of relaxation as an approach to everyday living*. Progressive muscular relaxation is usually carried out in a warm, darkened room with the clients lying on mattresses on the floor or on beds. Although this may be suitable in the initial stages of training, for effective results the acquired skills must be easily adaptable to everyday living. Therefore as the programme progresses, it is essential that the environment be normalised by admitting daylight and sound and allowing temperature fluctuations. Clients must also learn to achieve relaxation through cognitive control without the lengthy exercises used with the Jacobson method. They are encouraged to practise everyday activities in a relaxed manner by observing any unnecessary tensions and eliminating them.

7. *The acquisition of adequate coping skills*. Positive planning and reorganisation combined with reevaluation of operational and social skills are crucial. The client is encouraged to evaluate realistically and objectively previous non-coping behaviour and to note both the strengths and weaknesses. Role playing can provide a structured setting in which behaviour can be analysed with some accuracy and the literature of social skills provides useful analytical frameworks (e.g. Trower et al., 1978).

Role playing is valuable in that it provides the opportunity for rehearsal prior to facing a real life situation. The client may initially anticipate difficulty in approaching the role play seriously but usually becomes deeply involved. Acting out a situation reduces the anticipatory anxiety.

8. *The confrontation of alarming situations.* Gradual exposure to a feared object or situation has been an integral part of the treatment of phobias. The client is encouraged to relax whilst the stimulus causing the anxiety is gradually introduced. For example, animal phobias may be treated by introducing conversation related to animals followed by a photograph of an animal. Later, an animal skin or toy animal may be introduced and finally the real object of the client's fear.

If the subject of the phobia is less tangible, e.g. as in agoraphobia, a similar system of desensitisation can be used with the client talking about and imagining going out, followed by short trips, closely supervised, and eventually going out alone. The client is thus encouraged to face situations which he would normally avoid.

Setting up a group

Setting up an Anxiety Management Group is a cost effective method of treatment which may supplement drug-therapy or may be used as an alternative form of treatment. Recent studies have indicated that a significant proportion of clients have been able to substantially reduce or even cease their intake of medication during the course of treatment, although current trends aim to combine the best of each of these in a comprehensive approach to anxiety-based problems.

These methods allow one therapist to treat a group of up to six clients during each separate course which will equip them with a set of basic skills to enable them to adapt effectively to similar problem situations in the future. The techniques are easily taught by therapists with little psychological training, which may increase the availability of treatment.

Groups may be set up in the hospital, day centre or community to treat clients who are faced with problems due to their inability to cope with neurotic anxiety.

Selection of clients

Anxiety Management Groups should only be formed and incorporated as part of a departmental programme if there are clients referred for treatment who will benefit from the training. Too often, clients are included in a relaxation programme because that programme has become an integral part of the psychiatric department's treatment plan. Clients are selected to fill the available places in the group rather than a group being set up because the clients need it. Although this will not have a harmful effect to the client, it will not encourage the group-cohesiveness which plays such a major part in the development of the group. The common denominator in a correctly selected group of clients is that each member is unable to cope with his life because of neurotic anxiety which draws the group closely together and encourages the discussion of problems.

Clients are selected by interview for inclusion within a group and may be asked to fill out a questionnaire or a Mooney Problem Checklist before the meeting. This has two purposes; it causes the client to think about and to identify his particular problems, and allows the therapist to direct the interview using the information previously elicited from the questionnaire as she assesses his suitability for this form of treatment.

During the interview the client will be encouraged to talk about himself and his problems. He will be informed of the role he will be expected to play in the treatment programme and asked for his feelings about this proposal. He is made aware of the need for active participation and must demonstrate a willingness to attend the group sessions regularly.

Clients who are to be treated for agoraphobia at a day unit or in the community are expected to make their own arrangements to travel there. Ambulances are not ordered as this continues to reinforce the unwanted behaviour. The client is informed of this at interview and, although he may be apprehensive initially, as he plans how he will travel he will reduce his level of anxiety by the adoption of cognitive coping self-statements; for example, 'I could get my wife to bring me' or 'I will order a taxi'.

The agoraphobic client who accepts treatment under these terms has a good prognosis for recovery. He shows that he is willing to take the first steps in coping with his problems.

An analogy may be drawn to demonstrate to the client the role of the therapist and that expected from him. He is told of the patient who goes to his doctor with a sore throat and is given a prescription for antibiotics. This drug will cure his illness but he does not bother to take the prescription to the chemist or only takes the tablets for a few days rather than the prescribed course. His throat does not get better; in fact it may get worse and he goes back to his doctor to complain that he is still unwell. The doctor has no magic formula to help the patient. He can only diagnose the condition and provide the required treatment. The onus is on the patient for carrying out treatment. He cannot complain if he does not play his part as a member of a team. Likewise the responsibility for treatment rests with the client in the Anxiety Management Group. He is the most important member of the treatment team and only he can carry out the necessary tasks which will lead to recovery.

The therapist will teach him the necessary skills and will offer support but the client must play a more active role than in other forms of relaxation training. It is essential that this responsibility for treatment be indicated to the client at the initial interview.

The venue

The venue for the group should be a quiet, comfortable room with easy chairs which allow for support for the head. In the initial stages of training it is necessary for all external sources of interruption to be excluded by closing windows, drawing curtains and dimming lights. As the course progresses, the environment must be allowed to become as normal as possible with everyday noise, light and fluctuations of temperature admitted. This will allow the clients to practise the skills of arousal reduction in realistic situations.

The course

An Anxiety Management Training Course should have clearly defined stages and a beginning and an end, as with any planned treatment. If it is allowed to continue indefinitely, clients may become dependent on the group and may not attempt to use and develop skills as part of their everyday life outside of the department.

The course may be divided into distinct parts:
a. The introduction
b. Stage one relaxation
c. Stage two relaxation
d. Differential relaxation
e. Review and planning.

This allows for the therapist to decide over what period it will run and how many sessions of each stage are required. It is possible to experiment with different arrangements of the stages until a workable formula has been found that will suit both the needs of the clients and the availability of staff.

There must be continuity if the training is to be effective and, when staffing will allow, it is advantageous to have two therapists within one group to allow for cover if one should need to be absent. If a tape recording of the relaxation course is used, it will further allow for continuity of treatment because only the one voice will give instructions at the early stage.

a. *The introduction.* Clients are introduced to the course with an explanation of anxiety—what it is and how it works. They are encouraged to talk of their own problems briefly to allow the others to identify them with theirs. It is stressed that anxiety is not an illness but a natural defence mechanism and that the clients will play an active role in their treatment, unlike previous treatments some may have experienced, e.g. hypnosis.

It is usually necessary to explain that 'doing nothing' is not the same as relaxing. Many clients are unable to equate their problems with tension and will assert that they sit with their feet up and yet still feel the same symptoms of arousal. From the very beginning of the course they must be taught that it is possible to be doing nothing and to be tense, yet be carrying out an activity and be relaxed.

A record book should be kept from the first session. The client's names are entered and brief details of their problems as they see them. As the course progresses and the clients review the treatment and their progress, these details are included. It is important to reassure the client that the record is only for the group to review at the end of the course when it may be seen if goals have been achieved and benefit derived from the training.

b. *Stage one relaxation.* This stage is based on Jacobson's methods of progressive muscular relaxation. The clients actively tense specific muscle groups to the extreme level possible at a given verbal cue. The muscles are then relaxed and the client is instructed to observe the feeling of relaxation compared to that of tension.

Although many may feel more relaxed than they normally do this form of relaxation is difficult to carry out in a realistic situation.

c. *Stage two relaxation.* In stage two the client is introduced to the method of training which will allow him to cope with anxiety-provoking situations. The muscle groups are not actively tensed to help him to differentiate between the two states but he is asked to observe how much tension there is present in specific muscle groups at that time.

He then relaxes each group on the given cue until a feeling of deep relaxation is experienced. Occasionally, a client may fall asleep during this stage and must be gently aroused without disturbing the rest of the group. The purpose of the training is to adapt it to stressful situations, not to enable the client to sleep. He may, of course, use it to aid sleep in an appropriate situation, i.e. in bed.

At this stage the clients should be monitoring and recording their own levels of arousal and bio-feedback equipment may be introduced for those clients who cannot distinguish any change. Targets should also be set by the client, and the therapist must ensure that they are appropriate and specific.

d. *Differential relaxation*. The training practised in this stage will allow the clients to tense some muscles whilst keeping others relaxed. They will learn to walk without the whole body becoming rigid or tense. Many people use more energy than is necessary to carry out an activity, for example as when threading a needle. The whole body becomes tense as an attempt is made to pass the thread through the eye of the needle, when only the muscles of the upper limbs and the eyes should be active.

The clients will perform movements on cue whilst maintaining the relaxed state, and with practice will adopt them as an integral part of their everyday life.

e. *Review and planning*. Throughout the course clients will have been learning new skills and the appropriate application of them to their own lifestyle. They will also have learned to monitor and record their own observations of their physiological state. Targets will have been set and achieved and the client is then ready to use all the information wihout the direct support of the group.

At this time the clients and therapist will review and evaluate the total course, and the record book will be consulted to show how changes have been made as the course progressed. From this feedback of information the therapist may decide to amend the course for the next group.

The clients will be reminded of the other ways in which they can help themselves to remain calm and to cope with life. They can organise their day better and plan to allow adequate time for all activities including meals. Planning also allows for less uncertainty and therefore less stress.

Clients are encouraged to take up creative hobbies and to go out more. They are reminded that a return to their previous way of life will result in a return to their previous behaviour. Boredom and routine are often the worst enemies of the person under stress. Even changing the route to work occasionally can have a good effect on the outlook on life.

Clients will make specific plans for the future at this stage and this will be reviewed at a feedback session at some future date.

Suggested programme

A suitable arrangement of the different stages may be as follows:

Session 1
Introduction to the course
Talk on anxiety. Literature may be given for private reading
Questions and discussion
Session 2
Review of previous information given
Discussion of the components of anxiety and recording of symptoms
Introduction to relaxation
Session 3
Review of previous session
Stage one of the relaxation course
Session 4
Review
Introduction to biofeedback
Stage two relaxation
Session 5
Review
Stage two repeat
Set targets
Biofeedback
Session 6
Review
Stage two repeat
Biofeedback
Set targets
Session 7
Review
Differential relaxation
Discussion of target problems and strategies
Set targets
Session 8
Review

Differential relaxation
Role play
Set targets
Session 9
Review
Role play
Planning for the future
Questions and discussion
Date set for follow up.

Behavioural targeting

In the Anxiety Management Programme behavioural targetting is used as a method of identifying goals and of assessing progress. The targets are closely specified behavioural goals set by the client in consultation with the therapist. Vague therapeutic aims result in vague therapy. Clients who are asked what they would like to achieve from their treatment often say they would like to feel better. This is not specific enough to use as a goal and the therapist must help by pinpointing the targets which may be gradually reached in a graded method.

If a client wishes to go to the shops more often, the therapist must determine how often she goes at present. The client can then specify how often she wishes to go in future and with whom. The final target may then include some contingencies to allow for successful completion and may be thus: on Thursday January 4th and Saturday 6th I will go to the supermarket alone. I will leave home at 10.30 a.m. and buy all the items on my list. I will relax for 15 minutes before I leave home and will walk slowly in a relaxed manner. If I feel shaky I will stop at the coffee bar and relax until the feeling passes. If it is raining heavily I will set an alternative date.

Points may be awarded for each target met and a success score can then be calculated:

$$\frac{\text{(Points achieved} \times 100)}{\text{(Points possible)}}\ \%$$

If a client persistently fails to meet the goals he has set and it is certain that they are not too high, it will show that he is unwilling to actively participate in his treatment programme and it should be discontinued. He may be given a further set of targets to achieve and if he does so, treatment may be resumed.

CASE STUDIES

During 1979 a total of 177 day clients were treated at a Day Unit in the North West. A study of these clients revealed that the diagnoses were:

41 Anxiety and allied conditions

136 Non-anxiety based, e.g. schizophrenia, manic depression etc. Further analysis and assessment revealed that of the 136 'non-anxious' clients 54 were suffering from symptoms of underlying anxiety.

These 95 clients were taught the appropriate application of relaxation skills in Anxiety Management Training Groups and 80 continued to function in the community.

The following brief case studies are illustrative of the problems treated.

1st Client

Client: Nursing sister
Age: 31 years old
Diagnosis: Anxiety state

This client was living with her husband and was childless. She had not felt that she was an anxious person, but had developed an erythematous rash over her neck which caused her embarrassment. She was aware that the rash developed when she was subjected to stressful situations and accordingly she disguised it by wearing polo-neck jumpers, even in summer.

She gradually withdrew from social life, refusing even to go with her husband to visit family or friends. She could not give up her job but changed to a night duty on a geriatric ward to avoid difficult confrontations.

Eventually, she had to transfer to a day duty because of staffing difficulties and attended a case conference. When she had to give her report, she panicked completely and could not cope with the situation. She was sent on sick leave.

The client received relaxation training based on deep breathing exercises which she performed while lying on a bed in a darkened room. Although she could manage to reduce anxiety in this way, she could not do so in stressful situations.

She was referred to a hypnotherapist with little relief from symptoms and in October, 1979 was referred to a consultant psychiatrist on the team.

The aims of treatment were:

1. To reduce anxiety by teaching anxiety management techniques and by reinforcing the appropriate application of these skills in the day to day situations in the unit and in the community.
2. To increase confidence in social situations by teaching appropriate social skills involving the application of anxiety management techniques.
3. To give support and encouragement to the client and to help her return to work.

Stage 1

First attendance at Anxiety Management Group (AMG). Very apprehensive because of the number of patients attending the department. Avoided contact with other patients and staff and avoided any potentially anxiety-provoking situations.

Stage 2

Was surprised at the level of tension present before she began to relax. Set her first target—to go for a drink with her husband over the weekend.

Stage 3

Achieved her goal. Was still wearing polo-neck sweaters. Set a second goal to go for a drink where old friends would be.

By her eighth attendance she had set a target of decorating her mother-in-law's flat. She had had little contact with this very domineering woman for 12 months. She was also wearing open-necked blouses by this time.

Final attendance

Had achieved all her targets and went out for a meal to celebrate. At this time, the client was playing a more active role within the unit. She was elected to the patient/staff committee and was a valuable contributor in all activities.

The techniques she had learned were constantly put into practice and her behaviour reinforced verbally. Pressure was increased and her days of attendance reduced. On her days off, she was to attempt something constructive and these goals were precise.

Discharge

On 25th January, 1980, the client was discharged back to work. She saw her nursing officer before this date and arranged to work on clinics.

Follow-up

Out-patient appointments.

Continues to work well on clinics. Is no longer avoiding social situations and is able to give formal verbal reports without neurotic anxiety.

2nd Client

Client: Unemployed builder
Age: 45 years old
Diagnosis: Low back pain

The client had been a self-employed builder for a number of years. He injured his spine at L4/5 and was treated conservatively and by an accupuncturist with moderate relief.

When his mother-in-law became ill, he recognised that her problem was due to anxiety and when this was confirmed, he began to examine his own problem in this light. He attempted to relax but was unable to gain relief from low back pain.

He asked to be referred to a psychiatrist.

Aims of treatment

1. To reduce the level of anxiety by teaching appropriate A.M. Techniques.
2. To teach care of the spine in the work situation by showing the correct way to lift and bend.
3. To increase his confidence in his ability to produce a high standard of work by encouraging him to pass on skills to other patients.
4. To resettle in employment.

Stage 1

First attendance in A.M.G. Very apprehensive. Arrived by car as he was afraid of suffering incapacitating low back pain when out in public.

Coped with the initial exercises but was anxious about pressure on the lumbar spine.

Stage 2

Now sleeping well using A.M. Techniques. Discontinued nitrazepam.

Stage 3

Using public transport. Increasing walking time. Less afraid of injuring spine while in the community. Setting specific goals.

Final attendance

Now socialising and his confidence had increased. Great relief from low back pain.

The client continued to attend the unit but it was felt that he was becoming dependent on it. His days were accordingly reduced and he attempted to achieve further goals. He appeared to lack motivation in this direction, therefore a behavioural contract was drawn up in which he specified goals he wished to achieve. This would show both the client and the treatment team how well motivated he was.

The client failed to meet the requisite number of targets necessary for treatment to be continued and was discharged.

He continues to function well but misses the daily attendance at the unit. He is awaiting interview for a job with the local Council which involves inspecting houses in need of repair.

3rd Client

Client: Unemployed factory hand
Age: 32 years old
Diagnosis: Endogenous depression

This client worked in a local factory after leaving school until she was aged 21 years. She was engaged to be married to a man who was already married but had omitted to tell her.

She was informed by her workmates and broke off the engagement. She began to drink heavily and formed a relationship with a female workmate becoming heavily dependent on her.

Oue to remarks made by the client's colleagues and her possessiveness, the relationship ended and the excessive drinking increased. She suffered guilt feelings about her homosexuality and was afraid to face people she knew. She became very paranoid.

In 1968 she was admitted to the psychiatric ward via casualty after slashing her wrists. She refused to give a history and was diagnosed as depressive. She was treated with antidepressants and psychotherapy with little effect.

From 1968 to 1976 the client was admitted to the ward four times. She was attending occupational therapy on each admission but was uncooperative and restless. She was aggressive to both clients and staff. She was referred to the day unit when it opened in 1976 and travelled daily from home. There had been no change in her condition during the previous 8 years.

The aims of treatment

1. To reduce the level of anxiety by teaching A.M. Techniques.
2. To teach active coping skills and interactive social skills.
3. To teach the client to accept herself as she is without guilt feelings.

Stage 1

Refused to talk about her problems and insisted that she was not anxious. Sat on the edge of her chair wringing her hands. Rapid leg and foot movement noted. Participated in the exercises but had to get up immediately afterwards.

Stage 2

Was able to talk about her lack of confidence but not of her homosexual affair. Admitted to the fact that she was usually extremely tense and was now experiencing some relief.

Began to receive sexual counselling from the occupational therapist at this time as she refused to have any contact with the psychologists who were male.

She had begun to participate in other activities but avoided contact with male clients. Her contact with females was also limited as she was afraid that they may recognise her as a lesbian. Her occasional attention seeking and disruptive behaviour was modified at this time.

Stage 3

The client has now set targets which included shopping in an area where she was known and feared recognition. She achieved every target she set and was supplied with a tape recording of the A.M. Course in order for her to revise at a later date.

Because of her acquisition of relaxation skills, the client was able to join the social skills group and to date is forming appropriate relationships with clients and staff. She enjoys a quiet social life and is soon to leave the hostel where she lives for her own Council flat.

She is taking an interest in her appearance and is able to drink socially. She is aware that she has a cyclothymic personality and copes with mood swings by applying anxiety management techniques.

At the unit, she has been elected to the client/staff committee on three occasions. She has planned and taken activities with clients and used her training on these occasions. She is about to start an A.M. Group at the hostel and her days of attendance have been reduced. She hopes to find employment in the near future.

Her original diagnosis would seem inappropriate in retrospect. Many anxious clients present as depressives which may be due to their failure to meet goals they set themselves; the failure being due to neurotic anxiety.

SUMMARY

Anxiety is a normal defence mechanism which is designed to equip the body with increased energy in times of stress, whilst neurotic anxiety is a maladaptive response.

The treatment of anxiety with Anxiety Management Training is an active coping technique aimed at teaching clients to deal more effectively with the cognitive, physiological and behavioural aspects of anxiety. It is suitable for a wide range of clients, has no known adverse side-effects and may be used as a supplement or an alternative to medication.

Preliminary research suggests that the techniques, which are easy to learn, are valuable in a variety of settings. To date, treatment has been carried out in day units, psychology departments, activity units and in the community with both individual and group sessions.

In the physical field, therapists can use Anxiety Management Techniques to treat clients who are anxious about their disability, treatment or illness to cope in an appropriate manner. Often clients are discharged before the optimum level of recovery is reached because they are resisting treatment due to anxiety. By using this form of treatment anxiety can be overcome.

The greatest application for these techniques is in the field of health education and primary care. It is not necessary for an individual to wait until an anxiety problem has developed before benefiting from training. An improved ability to cope effectively with stress and tension will help both therapist and client to lead a happier, healthier life.

REFERENCES

Hittleman R 1971 Yoga for Health. Hamlyn, London
Jacobsen E 1938 Progressive relaxation. University of Chicago Press, Chicago
Miller R J, Cullen B, O'Brien R 1981 Are you sitting comfortably? Psychological approaches to the management of stress and anxiety. Occupational Therapy January: 5–9
Trower P, Bryant B, Argyle M 1978 Social skills and mental health. Methuen, London

RECOMMENDED READING

Barlow D H 1980 Patterns of desynchrony in agoraphobia. A preliminary report. Behavioural Research and Therapy 18(5): 441–448
Craighead L W, Craighead W E 1980 Implications of persuasive communication research for the modification of self-statements. Cognitive Therapy and Research 4(2): 117–134
Forsterling F 1980 Attributional aspects of cognitive behaviour modification: A theoretical approach and suggestions for techniques. Cognitive Therapy and Research 3(1): 27–37.
Grey S, Sartory G, Rachman S 1979 Synchronous and desynchronous changes during fear reduction. Behavioural Research and Therapy 17: 137–147
Jaremko M E 1979 A component analysis of stress inoculation; review and prospectus. Cognitive Therapy and Research 3(1): 35–48
Kirchner F, Stewart L, Shalett J 1978 Identification and management of the anxious patient within a model family practice unit. Journal of Family Practice (Mar) 6(3): 533–540
Ledwidge B 1978 Cognitive behaviour modification; A step in the wrong direction. Psychological Bulletin (Mar) 86(2): 353–375
Ledwidge B 1979 Cognitive behaviour modification; A rejoinder to Locke and Meichenbaum. Cognitive Therapy and Research 3(2): 133–139
Locke E 1979 Behaviour modification is not cognitive—and other myths; A reply to Legwidge. Cognitive Therapy and Research 3(2): 119–125
Meichenbaum D Therapist manual for cognitive behaviour modification. University of Waterloo, Ontario, Canada
Meyer V, Reich B 1978 Anxiety management—the marriage of physiological and cognitive variables. Behaviour Research and Therapy 16: 177

THE MANAGEMENT OF ANXIETY 181

Miller R J, Cullen B, O'Brien R 1981 Are you sitting comfortably? Psychological approaches to the management of stress and anxiety. Occupational Therapy January: 5–9

Miller R J 1979 Relaxation and the management of stress and anxiety (tape and information booklet). Psychological Counselling Services, 80 Rosemont Road, Liverpool L17 6DA

Miller R J 1979 Behavioural targetting. Unpublished manuscript

Richards C S 1978 When self-control fails: A case study of the maintenance problem in self-control treatment programs. Cognitive Therapy and Research 2(4): 398–401

Spielberger C D, Sarason I G (Eds) 1977 Stress and anxiety, Volumes 1–4. Hamisphere Publishing Corporation, Washington Halsted Press (John Wiley and Sons)

Spragg A K 1980 Anxiety management in General Practice: procedure and evaluation. M Psychol Dissertation, University of Liverpool

Suinn R M, Richardson F 1971 Anxiety management training: A non-specific behaviour therapy program for anxiety control. Behaviour Therapy 2: 498–510

Sutton-Simon K, Goldfried M R 1979 Faulty thinking patterns in two types of anxiety. Cognitive Therapy and Research 3(2): 193–203

Woodward R, Jones R D 1980 Cognitive restructuring treatment; a controlled trial with anxious patients. Behaviour Research and Therapy 18(5): 401–407

Creative therapies

INTRODUCTION

The term 'creative therapy' embraces the work of art therapists, music therapists, remedial dramatists, psychodramatists, movement and dance therapists. Here we describe the practice of creative therapy by occupational therapists. Although individuals may be treated by the methods outlined below, this chapter concentrates on group work.

The roots of creative therapy lie in psychoanalysis, Moreno's psychodrama and analytical psychology. It has developed alongside the 'Human Potential Movement', the underlying concepts of which were described in Chapter 4. Creative therapy has yet to identify its own discrete theoretical framework; its practitioners borrow their principles from psychotherapy and the study of group dynamics and their techniques from the arts, notably drama, movement, massage, dance, music, painting, sculpture, poetry and prose. The aim is to assist healing and 'personal growth' through active involvement in the expressive arts, within a psychotherapeutic group setting.

A creative therapy group operates as a miniature culture with specific rules of conduct which allow the participants a wider range of behaviours. This permits the socially unskilled to experiment with both self and others. For example, the tacit rules of dramatherapy allow touch, honesty, play, spontaneity, catharis and personal feedback. This may contrast with the culture in which the person became distressed, which perhaps insisted on diplomacy, decorum, inhibition, suppression and tact.

Some of the terms used within creative therapy illustrate the diversity of its origins. All participants, and not just the therapist, can be creative and so *transference* problems are diluted by placing emphasis on joint effort and the support of peers. Creative therapy groups provoke insight into unsatisfactory defense mechanisms

(Ch. 2) such as *repression, projection, denial* and *reaction formation.*
They encourage the anxious to *sublimate* basic drives in an acceptable way and *substitute* satisfying creative activities for those that are
socially unacceptable, for example, smearing clay rather than
faeces.

Personal potential may be realised where opportunity is provided
to express *shadow* traits, for example by evolving a dramatic role.
Group acceptance then facilitates the assimilation into the self of
these rejected parts, the process Jung described as *individuation.*
Finally, Reichs' concept of *character armour* which obstructs *lib-
idinal* energy is useful to therapists who encourage healthy posture
and expressive gesture in order to promote emotional release.

In the perplexing diversity and eclecticism of creative therapy lies
its greatest strength, for it provides a wealth of techniques and
media which are readily adaptable to individual needs and talents.
There should truly be something for everyone.

An occupational therapist, working through creative therapies,
will be hoping that members of the group can make gains in the
following areas:

a. Self-awareness and personal development.
b. The ability to express emotion in new ways where previous
   methods have been destructive either to oneself (e.g. drug and
   alcohol abuse, wrist cutting) or to others.
c. An understanding and exploration of problems within family
   relationships and other close or intimate friendships.
d. An awareness of problems experienced in initiating, developing
   and maintaining social contacts.
e. Insight into specific problems, for example, attitude toward
   authority figures.

The first section of this chapter looks at the skills and qualities
which the therapist needs to develop in order to lead creative
therapy sessions. This is followed by information about a selection
of media and their potential use, giving some examples of the type
of work which might be undertaken in sessions.

SKILLS AND ORGANISATION

The therapist

The first step is to involve oneself, as a participant, in different
types of creative therapy. Modes of expression differ, with personal
preference being given to a particular sense which will provoke

emotion. For example, some people in watching a film experience anger, sadness or happiness and may cry or laugh spontaneously. For these, visual stimulation is evocative of emotion; they may respond to art, pottery or visualisation techniques, such as working with dreams and fantasy. Others may find their emotions are more easily aroused by sounds. Music may comfort or scare them; they may be particularly vocal when excited and they may be open to techniques which involve listening to or making sounds using voices or instruments. Those who use their bodies to contact their emotions may release anger by hitting out, and experience happiness by dancing. Dance, movement, sport, mime and role play may be appropriate to their needs. Some use words and choose to write when they wish to express or to evoke feelings. These people may be drawn to creative writing, poetry writing and reading plays, verse or prose.

You may recognise which method is most appropriate to you, alternatively you may be lucky enough to be open to the use of several different media. If you are one of the latter, have patience with those amongst us who feel threatened or uninspired by some activities. Many of the patients will be limited in their emotional range and in their ways of expression.

Experience as a student

While on clinical placement you may be able to gain experience by joining groups which are run for patients. They may 'leave you cold' indicating that you are not currently open to that media or leave you feeling 'high and dry' having strong emotions which are not linked to anything. This may happen where you participate in a single session and cannot develop the feelings through regular participation, or where you are uncertain of your right to explore your feelings due to your membership of the staff team.

I feel that it is important to gain experience outside the thera-peutic setting. Sometimes this will occur on placements where there is opportunity to work in a student or staff group where you should be able to involve yourself fully in the experience, and make discoveries and changes for yourself. Outside the personal experi-ence, offered to you by college or by clinical placement, many workshops are run by different creative therapy organisations.

Personal skills and leadership

All therapists need to learn to use the 'self' as a tool within their work. This work will involve all types of personalities. There is increasing evidence to show that the relationship between therapist and patient is important if therapy is to be effective. In order to develop a trusting, warm, therapeutic relationship with patients it is necessary to understand yourself, to be aware of your own needs and limitations and to restrict yourself to using, within therapy, material with which you are familiar.

A summary of the qualities which a therapist needs to acquire is given below:

a. Self understanding, in terms of abilities, limitations, needs and sources of satisfaction.
b. Non-possessive warmth, genuineness and flexibility within relationships.
c. Basic personal security.
d. Knowledge of the dynamics of personal interaction.
e. Acceptance of each patient as an individual.
f. Experience, and an interest in expanding that experience.

The style of leadership which you adopt will be dependent on both your personality and on your intentions for the group. Many well known leaders in creative therapy are charismatic, that is they appear to inspire those around them and to impart energy to those with whom they are involved. However, it is possible to achieve effectiveness in a less central way. Good leadership occurs through the development of confidence in the methods being used and a manner appropriate both to yourself and to those who are being led. The following questions may be helpful when preparing and running sessions.

a. How much knowledge about the participants do I need before running the session?
b. Do I have sufficient confidence in the technique being used to enable me to focus my attention on the group members and their interactions rather than on practicalities?
c. Am I maintaining a balance between a directive and a non-directive approach in order to maximise the benefits, to the group and to individuals, of involvement and responsibility.
d. Am I in tune with people and responding appropriately to them?
e. Am I in tune with my own responses and behaviour within the session?

Co-therapy and supervision

One of the most effective ways to develop skills in leadership is to work, as a co-therapist, alongside an established therapist. You will be able to try out ways to enhance, intensify and moderate situations whilst receiving immediate feedback from a skilled person. Co-therapy is a partnership, and your own feelings and perceptions will be stimulating to the experienced leader, who may previously have been working alone and running risks of becoming stale or narrow.

It is important to obtain regular supervision from an objective outsider. The supervisor may be anyone who has the ability to help to identify and resolve difficulties. Peer group supervision can be useful; this involves being able to discuss feelings openly with colleagues. When specific difficulties arise the expertise from a wide range of disciplines can be drawn upon.

The more honest you can be within supervision, about the strengths and weaknesses of the session, the more helpful the supervisor can be. Part of the task of being a therapist using creative media is to remain open, to be willing to change, and to enjoy working in the sessions. A therapist who is bored and uninspired should take a break or move to a different area which offers a change of interest and stimulation.

The patients

Referral and assessment

Referral of patients may be the result of discussion by the whole team responsible for care both within and outside the unit. This may include the psychiatrist, psychologist, G.P., social worker nurses and occupational therapists. Some patients choose to refer themselves for this form of therapy. In some instances there is a specific request regarding difficulties which require to be worked on or technique to be used, in others the referral is left open and general.

The information that you will need to gather about each group member will vary with the aims of the group, the referring agency and with your own experience. The therapist usually meets each individual prior to them joining a creative group in order to initiate a relationship and to begin to understand how the patient relates to other people. If there is an opportunity to observe the patient in other settings, for example on the ward, in the occupational therapy department or within social groups, then the following features are of especial interest:

a. Responses to others. For example whether he is approachable, hostile, warm, withdrawn, liked or sensitive.

b. Responses to stress. When emotionally upset or confronted by others he may, for example, be accepting, unpredictable, aggressive, violent, sulky, communicative etc.

c. Evidence of some insight. Does the patient have an awareness both of his own mental state and that of others?

d. Evidence of internalisation. This is seen in an ability to take in, understand and learn from insight, and thus become open to change.

e. Any creative interests shown. Which general sessions attract him most? Does he attend, for example, musical activities in preference to those involving art?

From such informal observations as these, you should have some indication of an appropriate way to interview the patient and to introduce the idea of creative therapy. The initial approach will also depend on the patient's previous experience of therapy.

For patients who understand or have experienced creative therapy, or who have been referred by colleagues who are cognisant with creative approaches, the assessment interview will be straightforward. Aims can be established and a plan drawn up in order to work towards these.

For patients with limited experience of creative media, or those who have been referred with no specific indications about treatment, a fuller interview is necessary. Increasingly, occupational therapists use a problem-solving approach in which therapist and patient work together to list significant difficulties. The questions which they discuss include the following areas:

a. What problems are currently being experienced and what led up to them?

b. What kind of person is the patient, and what family and social relationships is he used to, now and in the past?

c. What does the patient want now and in the future? What are his expectations of therapy? What is his personal commitment?

From the list of problems drawn up, and from knowledge of the time span which is available or thought to be appropriate, a programme can be devised. Creative therapies will often be only a part of the treatment to be offered and will apply only to certain problem areas. The therapist should consider the individual's treatment programme as a whole and maintain close liason with other team members in order to ensure a coordinated approach and to monitor progress. By the end of the interview the patient should understand, as far as possible, the scope and potential of creative therapies without feeling too threatened. A further meeting should have been arranged to discuss and review plans and it should be clear that support and encouragement are available whenever required.

Before joining a group the patient may be invited to talk to appropriate existing members in order to gain some reassurance. All groups should be informed in advance of any new member who will be joining them.

Experience of change

The expectations that a patient has of treatment often includes an increased ability to cope, a feeling of well-being and happiness. It may be difficult for an individual to accept that experiencing difficult and uncomfortable feelings is the first stage in understanding and resolving issues which would have previously led to escapes such as food, drink, lethargy, drugs or disturbed behaviour. The second stage is to trust the therapist and the group to support, comfort and provide security while alternative ways of responding to past or present problems are found.

For individuals, progress can be recognised by reminding the patient of change through direct reference to his work, for example, by looking at a series of pictures or by repeating an earlier situation and pointing out changes in his responses. Patients will often acknowledge changes for themselves without requiring evidence Within a group, progress is usually obvious. At first, the group has no feeling of belonging or cohesion and people may express difficulties in sharing with the group and in trusting other members. As the group continues to meet, the depth of feelings being expressed increases, and with regular attendance relationships between members become increasingly close and warm. Members should start to show increasing abilities to take risks, to try out change and to express their fears and problems in the group. Finally, the patient will feel able to start changing in relation to people in the outside world, responding differently to stress situations. Within any therapeutic group the following processes should also be occurring:

a. Increased social contact through the integration of group members and relief from isolation.
b. Mirror reactions, where individuals begin to perceive themselves through the reactions of others.
c. Condenser phenomenon; this is the activation of the collective energy of the group which may intensify feelings.

d. Exchange, enrichment and feedback.

Types of group

The number of sessions planned and the level of work undertaken will be dictated mainly by the type of group. The two basic types of group are the 'closed' and the 'slow open'.

A closed group is one in which the same members meet for a predetermined number of sessions, new members do not join and members do not leave. The resulting consistent membership enables the group to work at an intense level. Careful selection of members is important, as is the size of the group which will largely determine the level on which it can work. Between five and eight members is the optimum size for groups working towards developing trust, self-disclosure and trying out new ways of expression. When working with larger groups it may be helpful to use split groups for part of the session. The composition of the group depends a great deal on your judgement. This should be based on a sound knowledge of group dynamics, a knowledge of your own relationship with each person and on observation of the way in which potential group members interact informally. It is usually helpful to have a group of fairly compatible people which includes a balance of personality types and of sexes.

A 'slow open' group holds regular, continuing meetings, with new members being introduced as others leave. People usually give notice of their departure, a decision which is subject to group influence. It may be that each member comes for a set number of sessions. I run a small psychodrama group which lasts for twelve weeks but consists of three sections, each of four weeks, when members may leave or join. Some people are very unwilling to open themselves to creative therapies, I feel that any strong resistance should be respected.

Basic organisation

The venue

The following points should be considered when choosing a room:

a. *Size.* The room should be appropriate to the number of people in the group so that members are neither 'lost' in the area available nor invading each other's personal space. 'Body work' requires approximately two square metres per person where there is to be free movement or work involving rolling or lying on the floor.

b. *Availability*. Ensure that the chosen room is available on the days and at the time required, allowing for preparation and tidying up. Conference rooms, gyms, dance halls and dining rooms can be used for movement and large drama groups, providing permission is obtained.

c. *Freedom from interruption*. Ensure that, through liaison with colleagues and through clear notices, the session will not be interrupted by the telephone, by people passing through or by people looking in through windows or doors. Curtains can be drawn to exclude the rest of the world but this can make those outside inquisitive, and those inside feel that they are involved in something clandestine.

d. *Suitability*. For movement and drama sessions where work is often done in a circle, a square room rather than a long, thin one should be chosen. Floor covering is important and a carpeted or smooth surface may be essential. Mats may occasionally be satisfactory. The furniture in the room may be unsuitable. If necessary, ensure that it is easy to move, that you have permission to move it and that it can be moved to an appropriate place where it does not block a fire exit.

For music sessions seating may be needed for listening to music or for playing. Suitable storage space must be found for equipment and electrical sockets available if required. If equipment is to be kept away from the occupational therapy department check on the security arrangements and insurance. For art and creative writing make sure that there are suitable seats and working surfaces and that space is sufficient to make paints, paper and water accessible nearby.

Always leave any room suitably arranged for the next occupants.

e. *Accessibility*. You should consider the distance to be travelled to the room, the transport of materials and equipment, water and toilets and general ease of location for group members.

Timing of sessions

The duration of sessions should be decided by considering the patients' total programme in relation to the emotional depths and stresses likely to be experienced in the group. With intense groups, such as 'projective' art and psychodrama, try to avoid times immediately before weekends, after small group psychotherapy (unless you are able to modify the session accordingly), and before or during ward rounds and case conferences. The length of each session will vary but, for practical reasons, should be seldom less than an hour or more than two hours.

Problems of non-involvement

All therapists at some time or other, face the problem of a creative therapy session that fails to work. These sessions can be used in a constructive way to develop the therapist's skills of leadership. They emphasise that the support of a co-therapist and a supervisor is crucial to keeping the situation in perspective. Some common problems are summarised here.

Poor relationship between the therapist and a patient

Possible reasons include:
a. You remind him of someone about whom he has intense feelings.
b. He reminds you of someone about whom you have intense feelings.
c. Your approach or manner is at fault. You are too interpretative, not interpretative enough or insufficently trusted.
d. You appear to like some patients more than others.
e. You are detected as having a lack of confidence in the technique being used.

The solution may lie in discussing the problem openly, exploring all the possible reasons for the difficulties and the ways in which these may be resolved.

Poor relationships between group members

Possible reasons include:
a. They feel that they do not know each other.
b. They do not like each other.
c. There have been arguments or disagreements outside the group.
d. One member particularly upsets the group and becomes a scape-goat for all the group's difficulties.
e. Two people are seen as working together, both inside and outside the group, to expose individual and group vulnerabilities.
f. Group members are not attending consistently.

The solutions are as varied as the sources of the problem. Try to deal with these by structuring discussion within the group. Allow time for group members to get to know each other and for feelings to be dissipated through some indirect channel. Discuss the problems of being a 'scapegoat' or an outsider in the context of groups and belonging. Explore the security and power of being part of a pair and the exclusiveness which this implies. Examine, with the group, any problems of attendance.

Inappropriate media or techniques

Possible reasons include:
a. Poor referral or assessment.
b. The technique used is too superficial or too deep for the group's capacity at the time.
c. Bad timing or arrangement of the session, insufficient warm up or preparation of individuals.

The solution may be to spend more time working out aims for the group and exploring relevant media. Advice may be sought from colleagues and the ways in which individuals are prepared for the group revised.

Hostility from outside the group

This problem may be identified when participation in the group's activities is discouraged by other patients, staff or friends and relatives.

Possible solutions include providing a more coherent explanation of creative therapies to each group stressing the reasons for inclusion or exclusion and discouraging bizarre interpretations of what is happening. If the difficulty lies within staff relationships, more time should be given to improving communication and to giving more information about the progress of each patient who is involved.

Other problems arising from the environment or from the patient's commitments to other activities should be resolved by attending more thoroughly to organisational details.

MEDIA USED WITHIN CREATIVE THERAPIES

Drama

Drama implies activity and has come to include a wide range of techniques. These involve role play, and trust, sensitivity and encounter work (TSE). TSE consists of exercises which increase people's awareness of themselves and of their interaction with others, both verbally and non-verbally. They may be used on their own or as an integral part of a session involving role play. Role play is also used in psychodrama and, incidentally, in social skills training.

Clarification of terms

a. *Social drama*. A fairly informal role play, usually encompassing social situations.

b. *Sociodrama*. The use of role play to explore problems common to the group members. For example, an adolescent group may role play difficult situations at home.

c. *Psychodrama*. This is the most intimate of the role playing techniques. Psychodrama is the exploration of a situation specific to one individual in the group, although others will often relate to the situation. The session will usually evoke, in the individual whose role play it is, the emotions involved at the time of the given situation. The therapist therefore aims to help the patient express these emotions satisfactorily. Psychodrama is often a powerful experience for all those involved and should be treated with both caution and respect. For this reason I feel strongly that the inexperienced should steer clear of it, and hence I will not be describing it in any great detail.

The selection of patients

a. *Social drama*. This may be used with all types of patients. It is however advisable to gather together those with similar needs.

b. *Sociodrama*. Careful selection of patients is advised in order to produce a balanced group. It is wise to involve people who will bring pressure to bear on individuals to respond within the social norms appropriate to their background and culture. Do not include many people with aggressive or psychopathic tendencies.

c. *Psychodrama*. Some patients are unsuited to exploring their problems through psychodrama. This is because it involves gaining insight into their own problems while having sensitivity to those of other group members. It is often wiser to exclude newly admitted patients and those in an acute state of illness. Likewise, dementing patients, actively suicidal patients and those who are suffering borderline psychotic states should not be considered. The middle-aged patient who clings rigidly to convention in order to cope may not benefit from the technique, and similarly patients in advanced and deteriorating organic states, those who have an alcohol or drug dependence and those patients who are over anxious ought not to be included.

For the patients mentioned above, there may be a danger of the precipitation of acting out symptomology through psychodrama.

d. *Trust, sensitivity and encounter exercises*. These may be modified to suit almost all groups of patients. TSE exercises provide a structure and a boundary allowing touch between people, a thing many patients may not have experienced for some time.

The organisation of drama sessions

Any session taking place may be divided up into three parts.

a. The warm-up period during which you prepare the individual or group for the task to be done. Preparation may be verbal, for example a discussion or expression of feelings, or non verba, perhaps using movement or the exploration of sounds, rhythms or gestures. A combination of verbal and non-verbal techniques may be used.

b. The 'core' or role play time is used for exercises which explore areas upon which the group is focussing. This part of the session may allow new ways of seeing a problem to be uncovered, or may allow the expression of previously suppressed emotions. This may involve the risk of personal disclosures through both verbal and non-verbal communication. All group members should be involved in this part of the session.

c. The 'wind-down time', or end of the session is crucial. It may include discussion, relaxation and tension reducing exercise.

Timing

Both 'warm-up' and 'wind-down' periods should last from five to fifteen minutes each. The 'core' of the session should range from thirty to sixty minutes duration. It is important not to skimp on either 'warm-up' or 'wind-down' time as the group members may find it difficult to adapt to and from the core exercises. Respecting the time limits of a group is important as members will feel more secure if they know the length of a session and will be less likely to leave a stressful exercise when they know that time is limited.

Examples of techniques used within core exercises

a. *Sculpting*. This is a versatile technique which uses people as 'models' and 'sculptors'. For example, with the group working in pairs, one person sculpts the other into perhaps the expression of an emotion. The whole group may then compare and discuss the different ways in which the emotion has been depicted. Alternatively, one person may sculpt the whole group into one tableau to express an emotion. Progressing from this, and particularly in small, well-established groups, an individual may sculpt other group members into a representation of his family's emotional relationship. Physical distance between sculpted individuals may, for example, represent the emotional difference between family members.

b. *Role reversal*. This technique may give an individual insight into the feelings others have about his behaviour or may give a fresh perspective on a situation. For example, adolescents may take parental roles and older group members adopt the persona of an adolescent. This is a technique used by some family therapists.

c. *Egoing or doubling*. Here the therapists or another group member may intervene to help a participant who is at a loss for words or action. Observers take advantage of feeling that they know what a participant ought to do or say next, stepping into the role play and temporarily taking on an individual's part. The usual method is to rest a hand upon the shoulder of the individual for whom you wish to speak, to say your piece and then to step aside again. The hand on the shoulder of the participant indicates to him that he is being spoken for and he continues the role play as soon as the hand is removed from his shoulder.

d. *The use of symbols*. The use of symbols is widespread throughout drama and the other creative therapies. For example, the group or individuals may describe themselves or others as animals. This exercise may then be extended by the acting out by individuals of the animal roles ascribed to them.

Alternatively a form of 'twenty questions' may be used. Here the group attempt to identify an individual through various symbols. For example, to the question, 'What type of tree would this person be?' the answer may be 'An oak'. Once identified, the individual concerned may reflect upon whether he recognises himself, and upon his reactions to the descriptions of him.

These exercises allow individuals to express things they notice about themselves and others in an indirect way. Most people find this far less threatening than a confrontation. The willingness to express the self symbolically is often a step towards direct verbal sharing. For example, the person within a group who seems strong and unapproachable may be symbolised as a lion. When asked how he would respond when on his own, or how he would like to respond, he may curl up or offer a tentative paw. It may then be possible to explore the emotions symbolised verbally.

e. *Empty chair.* This is a powerful technique in psychodrama which is often used in a modified way. An empty chair is used to depict people for whom unresolved feelings need to be explored by an individual. These feelings may be positive or negative. The empty chair is frequently used in coping with grief. The technique may be used prior to family or marital sessions in order to release feelings, and it may help those individuals who fear role play or are embarrassed by the thought of offending others who are also playing parts.

Trust, sensitivity and encounter work

The dictionary definition may guide us to an understanding of the aims of TSE work. Trust is defined as 'worthiness of being relied on, confidence in the truth of anything'. Encounter is described as 'to meet face to face' and sensitivity as 'feeling readily capable of receiving stimuli'.

Exercises and techniques have been evolved to help the individual develop, experience, and recognise non-verbal messages, needs, and abilities, incorporating them with the appropriate verbal meassage. Some way in which work may progress are mentioned below.

Allowing ourselves to fall and to be caught by others emphasises the problems of developing trust. Working in pairs, partners are asked to face each other, one becoming 'the trusting' and the other 'the trusted'. Initially, the trusted partner supports the trusting individual by placing both hands on his shoulders and taking the weight as the trusting partner gradually leans forward. The amount of weight taken by the trusted is gradually increased. The leader of the group encourages the partners to try to gauge with sensitivity, and without speaking, how far the trusting partner wants to go and how far the trusted feels safe to take the trusting individual. A compromise between the two partners is reached. Having worked in silence, the pairs then examine verbally how both felt before changing roles. Over numerous sessions, partners will find themselves increasingly able to trust and may even be able to allow themselves to fall and be caught.

As an addition to this work, an exercise known as 'the pivot' may be used. Within a group of six to eight people, one person elects to stand with the rest of the group around him, all, initially, with their hands upon him. The group members become the trusted and the central individual the trusting, allowing himself to be supported in any direction. In this exercise the group must be sensitive both to the central individual and to each other. The therapist may pose questions relating to the trust felt, for example, 'Does this reflect your degree of comfort with a group rather than with an individual?' or 'How did you feel about having to take responsibility for another person?' Once the group has established that these exercises relate to their responses in personal and social life then such questions will no longer be needed.

Art

Free unstructured sessions

Time is given for people to work in whatever way they wish. Talking informally with people, the therapist will find that most of the pictures will reflect something of the person's current feeling and will often say something about their past or future.

Depressed and despairing patients may paint messages to indicate how they feel, psychotic patients may depict their hallucinations or the way in which they feel confused and out of control. Suicidal patients may indicate their intention and lonely patients their need to talk about their feeling of isolation.

Guided sessions with an informal group

a. *Use of music.* Music can be used to trigger off feelings and ideas in individuals. One piece of music or series of pieces can be used and one picture or series of pictures composed. Individuals may work independently, the group may work together on a single sheet, or in a form of 'consequences' with the picture moving on with each change of music. Following the painting time, the group can share the different emotions and memories the music evoked.

b. *Task oriented work.* A group may work together to produce a particular piece of work that may vary from a practical project, for example, designing posters or cards, to more insightful projects such as producing posters advertising the skills of the group, or sharing a large paper to design a house for the group with each individual having his own ideal room.

c. *'Projective' art groups.* This is usually a slow open or closed group of six to ten people who meet regularly. They may or may not have similar problems, but they should function at a similar level of ability to use abstract thoughts and to be capable of insight. The group may decide on a topic or the therapist may provide one. Topics may cover a wide range, for example, 'me in the family', leaving hospital, freedom, dependence, awareness, parents. The group should paint for 20–40 minutes, depending on the time available and the capacity of the patients. The group is encouraged to spend the painting-time in silence, thinking of the topic and using the paints in whatever way they like. Symbols may be used, a whole scene painted, words used, pin figures or absolutely anything that the painter finds useful to depict feelings, ideas and experiences. Members of the group are encouraged to remain in the room with their painting even if they feel they have finished early. Often the feelings evoked by the topic are difficult ones to cope with and this may lead to a desire to leave. Following the painting period, each member of the group shows his painting and shares as much as he wishes to what he has depicted on the paper and of the feelings which the topic evoked. Over a series of sessions the group will become able to point out themes in an individual's work and to encourage each other to reveal deeper conflicts and feelings hinted at within the pictures. I usually say that each person is at liberty not to answer questions or to be drawn on a point by the group and this helps individuals to paint freely during the painting time. I find each painting needs five to ten minutes spent on it, the amount of time increasing as members of the group get to know each other better.

Projective art groups can be used in conjunction with group and individual psychotherapy, with patients being encouraged to try out expression in the art session as a prelude to expressing material verbally in the group or individual setting.

Most therapists work as a leader/participant in projective art. This enables the therapist to act as a model, and to develop a giving and taking relationship with the group rather than an authoritarian role.

As a guide to new therapists who are worried about how open to be, I suggest that in the first group they behave, like any newcomer, with caution.

When a topic evokes strong emotion in a therapist she should try to find a way of indicating the feelings without focussing on the group's attention on herself. For example, after a divorce the topics of 'separation', and related ideas could evoke overwhelming feelings that may not be hidden. At the discussion time she may begin by saying something like: 'This topic has been hard for me to paint because the emotions that it evokes are painful for me and it is a problem which I am currently trying to resolve.' This statement would allow her to share her feelings while stating that the problem was not for open discussion.

Art with individuals

Some people need to work on a one-to-one level. They may have problems that are specific to them and need to be worked at individually. They may need to have some individual sessions to learn how the use art before joining a group. They may be sufficiently sensitive and vulnerable that the extra support, and directed attention, of the therapist is needed. In the context of individual work the therapist may not always participate. it being inappropriate for the therapist to expose her own problems. Alternatively, the therapist may work alongside the person with the aim of establishing rapport.

Finally art is part of treatment and as such it may be used directly to feed back to the rest of the team at meetings and ward rounds. It is important to make it clear to the patients that this may happen.

Creative writing

As with art and drama, creative writing can apply to any number of writing and reading activities used by occupational therapists to help people recognise their potentials and explore problem areas.

Writing as a way of expression has several advantages:
a. Intellectuals often feel more secure when given the opportunity to use words.
b. People who are too threatened by paints may use writing.
c. It provides a record of feelings.
d. It provides an opportunity to experiment with the verbal expression of feelings.
e. Reading out what has been written helps people to admit their feelings and to gain confidence.

Creative writing in some form is suitable for anyone who can read and write. It should be ensured that everyone attending the session can do so.

Guided sessions with an informal group

a. *Poetry writing group*. The group is provided with materials and space for writing. The group may all decide to write on the same theme, a limited selection of themes or individually.

A time is given for the writing, and then the work is read out.

It should be an understood expectation that work will be read out and that members can help each other to gain confidence in reading their own work or allowing another person to read it. In a 'one-off' group it is understandable that there may be reluctance to read what has been written; as an alternative an outline may be given.

b. *Writing with music*. Music can be used to provoke feelings and memories during a writing session.

c. *'Poetry consequences'*. This is a useful introduction to using writing creatively and may give people confidence in their abilities. Each person writes a title for a poem or contributes the first line. The papers pass around the group, each person adding a line to what has previously been written. After the poems are completed they are read out. Poems created in this way usually reflect the overall mood of the group and give a sense of cohesion.

d. *Poetry or story completion*. This can be used for people who are too threatened by pen and paper to write anything. A few lines of a poem, or the opening paragraphs of a story, are given to each person or to each pair and time allowed for this to be taken to some conclusion. Once completed the stories are shared.

e. *Play writing*. As a group project this can be taken to a variety of levels. A group could work independently on short, imagined dialogues between people. This could build up to producing a review or a play for performance. Producing a play incorporates most of the creative therapies and hence nearly everyone could find a niche, with help and guidance from the therapist.

f. *Story writing*. Through a story, which uses imaginery characters, individuals will often share secret parts of themselves quite unconsciously.

g. *Poetry/prose reading*. Although this does not involve writing, poems and prose that individuals enjoy can be brought to a group to be read. Discussion of why the individual enjoys the poem, the author or the style and the feelings evoked by the poem for other group members helps individuals to express themselves. It forms a good warm-up activity or helps people to make their own contribution.

h. *Guided sessions with a closed or slow open group.* People write either freely or upon fixed topics for 20–30 minutes followed by a period of sharing of individual work.

Music

Music can be taken to include creation of sounds and tunes; the use of voice and the listening and sharing of music. The advantages of music as a creative medium within therapy include the following:

a. The activity may be very simple, for example, developing rhythms as a group.
b. Music may allow the expression of pent-up energy using either instruments or voices.
c. Verbal skills and intellectual ability are not necessarily needed.
d. A piece of music can express an individual's feelings without the necessity of making a personal statement.
e. Music may be a passive activity.
f. Feelings can be evoked through the external stimuli provided by a piece of music.

Ways of sharing music

There are many ways in which people can coordinate their interests in sounds and music. On a simple level, sessions can be reserved for individuals to bring to the group pieces of music which have particular personal meaning. Those who have instrumental skills may offer performances or basic instruction to encourage others to join in.

Many people find difficulty in producing noise; sessions that aim to develop the ability to shout or sing freely should be treated with sensitivity. It may be helpful to discuss the origins of inhibitions about creating noisy sound; individuals may recall being shouted at in a threatening way or associate screaming with being out of control or with other fears. Gradually building up freedom from inhibition can help to increase the ability to express a range of feelings, in particular the release of anger and frustration. Combining the use of the voice with the production of instrumental sound often allows freer vocal expression.

Singing is a more structured activity than 'sound-making' but gives a group cohesion and allows individuals to gain ascendancy to initiating ideas.

Music can be used as an inspirational source within other creative activities, such as art, writing, movement or pottery, thus encouraging creativity and expression within the individual.

Body work

There is an increasing interest in the link between body and mind. This is reflected in society by the growing emphasis on sport, body care and fitness programmes which include such activities as jogging, exercise machines and classes in yoga, T'ai Chi, aerobics and expressive dance. Keep fit, sport and some forms of dance and movement and relaxation have traditionally been part of occupational therapy programmes. These are usually group activities in which the majority of patients participate, the overall aim being to increase fitness, encourage awareness, reduce tension and develop greater freedom in range of movement. A direct link was not always made between these activities and psychological well-being. This view is changing and many therapists have sought further experience and training for themselves.

Many therapists have developed considerable skills in bioenergetics, contact release, aerobics, yoga, mime, gestalt methods, Laban and other approaches. They use their own experience and their special knowledge to take a wide variety of group and individual sessions. Such knowledge can be acquired by both reading and by attending appropriate courses.

Application

Those whose body image or awareness is distorted, for example those with obese, anorexic or bulimic problems, may benefit from this medium as may those whose movements have become stiff, restricted and tense. These include, for example, those with acute anxiety states and depressed states. Those who are self-conscious and embarrassed by their bodies, and those who find it difficult to express themselves verbally should also find body work to be helpful.

Some examples of work involving the body

a. *Relaxation and guided fantasy.* Using a simple relaxation technique to prepare the group, the leader then takes the group on a fantasy journey. The journey always begins and ends in the room in which the session is taking place. Each person becomes involved in their own thoughts and ideas during the fantasy trip. Afterwards, the feelings and ideas produced can be depicted on paper, in words or in movement and shared in small groups. This is an evocative technique and the patients should be carefully chosen. Generally, the precautions for psychodrama apply.

b. *Relaxation and body awareness.* Through the modification of relaxation techniques a group can be directed to concentrate all their thoughts on each part of the body in turn. This technique may help patients become aware of parts of their body that they neglect, or which are tense or over used. This may be a useful preparation for movement sessions.

c. *Warming-up the body.* Keep fit and sport are one way to do this. Freedom is given to individuals to use ideas evolving from stretching, dropping, uncurling the spine, falling and balancing, working alone, with partners and in groups. The leader must stress the importance of each individual working for themselves within their own limits without becoming concerned with the activity of others.

d. *Movement using themes.* Themes may be developed in many ways. Here are two ideas:

(i) *Contrasts.* Moving with opposites first one way then in another, for example, openness and concealment, freedom and restriction.

(ii) *Time in the past.* Each person recalls a time or experience from their past and moves in the manner appropriate to that period.

Pottery

Clay has an ancient history in psychiatric treatment and in most hospitals you will find a pottery department. Many patients will attend pottery to develop skills and to produce traditional coil pots, thumb pots and thrown vessels, often taught by a pottery technician. The resulting work may increase self-esteem. Clay can be used in a less structured way for the expression of feelings. Watching people with clay, you will find them playing with it, rolling it, shaping it, moulding it, pushing their fingers and fists in it, stretching it and, almost always, becoming thoroughly absorbed in the activity.

Application

A group may work together to produce shapes, imaginary figures and animals which may be brought from their dreams, fantasies or hallucinations. Music may be used to stimulate ways of playing with the clay. Soft gentle music giving soft gentle movements, strong angry music may lead to slapping the clay into the bench etc. In this way the clay is used as a recipient of feelings and may not be moulded into any form at all. People who are unwilling to communicate with others may be able to be reached through clay during individual sessions. Both therapist and patient can work alongside each other to create forms and express feelings.

RECOMMENDED READING

Alvin J 1966 Music therapy. Baker, London

Blackner H 1973 Acting. In Practical applications of psychodynamic methods. Springer Publishing Company, New York

Houston G 1976 All in the mind. BBC Publications, London

Houston G 1982 The relative sized red book of gestalt. The Rochester Foundation, London

Jennings S (ed) 1975 Creative therapy. Pitman Books, London

Jennings S 1973 Remedial drama. Pitman Books, London

Ryecroft C 1968 A critical dictionary of psychoanalysis. Nelson and Sons, London

Storr A 1972 The dynamics of creation. Secker and Warburg, London

Wethered A 1973 Movement and dance in therapy. MacDonald and Evans, London

10

Margaret Nichol

Constructive activities

INTRODUCTION

Everyone uses activity. Through activity we test our knowledge, relate to each other, practise or learn skills, experience fun or pleasure, express feelings and achieve control over our lives. The unique characteristic of occupational therapy is the use of carefully planned activity as a treatment medium. 'Constructive activities' are included within strategies which can be used with short-term psychiatric patients.

Constructive activities include the broad heading of work, self-care and social and recreational learning through participation. There are two main aspects of constructive activities:
1. The greater understanding of self
2. The development of skills

Both are interdependant; one area is not seen as being more important than the other. Within treatment some activities are structured to provide self-understanding while others produce improved skills. Constructive activities may occur in groups or on a one-to-one basis. However, due to pressure of time, and because people live and function in groups, they are commonly used with small groups of patients. Group dynamics occur in any group, including groups using constructive activities, and the occupational therapist must be able to recognise these and to use them to the patients' advantage. It is not the major purpose of this book to discuss group dynamics, therefore students should also refer to a book on this subject. In order for the occupational therapist to function in these groups she must understand both herself and also what a well-integrated person can do and feel.

Using this knowledge the occupational therapist can help the patient to determine where problems lie and the possible solutions that are available.

205

Constructive activities produce the following:

1. Information is gained about the patient through observation of his participation in the various activities. This may include his ability to relate to others and to you, his present degree of skill, his ability to concentrate, his motivation and manual dexterity.
2. Self-esteem can be developed by the patient through gaining more information about himself from others in the group and through achieving success and more confidence while involved in activities.
3. New skills can be acquired.
4. Activities can be used to channel emotional needs, for example the experience of cathartic release.
5. Specific cognitive deficits can be improved.
6. New interests and skills can be developed for use after discharge, when the patient needs to become re-integrated into the community.
7. A degree of structure and organisation is provided which is useful to many patients and through which they can participate, initially, at a comfortable level.
8. The provision of a way of focussing on the practical aspects of the 'doing' process. This may help individuals who have problems in actually engaging in activity rather than just talking about it.
9. The provision of a means of measuring the patient's progress. The patient can measure achievement and progress in terms of the activity.

ACTIVITY ANALYSIS AND PROGRAMME PLANNING

Analysing activities and planning appropriate programmes are essential in order to relate to the functional and personal needs of the patients. Before an occupational therapist can analyse an activity or plan a programme for a patient she should consider the following:

1. The patient—specific factors: e.g. age, sex, previous/present occupation, social background, diagnosis, prognosis, any physical disabilities, interests, approximate intellectual level.
2. The environment, e.g. facilities available: woodwork shop, domestic unit, pottery, gym, etc.; equipment available: audio-visual aids, art materials, sports equipment, etc.; staff available: helper, technical instructor, pottery technician, etc.; position in environment—rural or urban etc.

3. The therapist: e.g. knowledge, skills, personal interests, level of experience and creativity etc.

Having built up a picture of what type of activities could be available to her the occupational therapist should now analyse each and identify their respective parts and demands. The first part should involve breaking down the activity and should identify:

1. The environment, facilities for individual activity.
2. The time required for completion.
3. Whether it can be modified to make it more complex or easier.
4. The more complex skills which are required to perform the activity.

The last point must be examined in greater depth and consideration should be given to the following:

1. Interpersonal/social demands

Does the activity require the sharing of ideas or tools etc? Does the patient have to interact in a verbal or non-verbal way? Does the patient need to cooperate or to be responsible to others?

2. Independence/dependent demands

Does the patient need to make decisions, take iniative, plan and organise, rely on others?

3. Cognitive demands

Does the patient need to make decisions, take initiative, plan and organise, rely on others?

4. Physical demands

Does the activity require strenuous activity, what type of motor movements are required, what senses are used?

5. Emotional demands

Is the activity stimulating, boring, repetitive, etc?

The above is not an all-inclusive list and readers should read more comprehensive descriptions of the analysis of activities in other books and journals.

When planning programmes for patients each must have a

programme which will cater for his individual needs. We all have basic needs; they can be described broadly as:

1. The need for self-preservation.
2. The need for social interaction.
3. The need to contribute to society.

Therefore, the occupational therapy programme should be broadly based on these three needs and should include work, social and domestic/self-care activities.

Obviously, not all these three aspects apply to everyone. Someone who is retired will require less emphasis on work but will possibly require more help in socialising and feeling that he can contribute to society, for example through contributing in some voluntary capacity.

Therefore, each of these three broad areas, work, domestic/self-care and social/recreational activities, will be considered separately. Care must be taken not to compartmentalise these activities as many of them fulfil several functions; for example a beauty group may fulfil a self-care or a social function.

WORK-RELATED ACTIVITIES

Many patients now attending short-term units are unemployed due to the present economic recession. This requires the occupational therapist to re-orientate her thinking about work and work-related activities—many patients, no matter how much they may want to work, will not do so again. It is unlikely that full employment will ever be achieved and the days of a high percentage of unemployment are with us. An occupational therapist must bear this point in mind when planning programmes for individual patients. She must be aware of the current employment situation in her area and decide accordingly whether or not it is appropriate to place patients on a work-orientated programme. Other factors which may influence her are: (a) the patient's age—if he is young then it may be more appropriate to instil some hope of working than if the patient is nearing the age for retirement; (b) work skills that patients have and whether these an be utilised in other work areas; (c) other potentials for employment in the area.

The occupational therapist must be realistic in planning programmes as it can be psychologically damaging to patients to instil hope of achieving if this is obviously not possible. Another factor which may adversely affect a patient's chances of getting job is the stigma associated with psychiatric illness. Many patients feel this quite acutely and require help to overcome it. Social skills training, or sociodrama, which are dealt with in other chapters of this book, are the usual way of dealing with job interviews and with situations which demand some explanation of the patient's psychiatric history.

Assuming that a patient is already in a job, or that the job prospects are good, the occupational therapist must, as part of the programme, introduce work-related activities. This can be done gradually by involving the patient in progressive activities which should help build up, for example, concentration, memory, manual dexterity, initiative, stamina and interpersonal relationships, all of which are usually required to function in a job. Following this, or as an alternative, the patient may be placed in a work unit where an assessment can be carried out and work habits reinforced. These work units vary and may involve clerical work, industrial/factory work, heavy manual work or catering/domestic work. Placements in the appropriate unit will depend upon the patient's previous work skills, and the expressed work preference, plus the vacancies that may exist within these units.

The occupational therapist working in the short-term unit must liaise with the staff of such units, whether occupational therapists or others, to ensure that the patient achieves the maximum potential advantage. The occupational therapist must inform the work rehabilitation unit staff about the patient and what the requirements are, for example, assessment or retraining in specific areas. She must also indicate what the discharge plans are and what part the work unit staff will be expected to play. She must report back to the rest of the ward team on the patient's progress in the work placement and indicate, if it is appropriate, when the patient is meeting with the Disablement Resettlement Officer (DRO). The DRO will help the patient to find employment or advise on Employment Rehabilitation Centres (ERC) which the patient may attend for a further assessment. He can also advise on the government retraining schemes available.

If the patient is returning to a job it may be necessary to liaise with the employer. This may be done either by the occupational therapist or the social worker or both. This may be necessary to assess the demands of the job the patient will be doing so that this can be simulated, if possible, within the hospital. This is particularly relevant when treating schizophrenic patients whose abilities may have deteriorated due to the illness and who therefore may not be able to function at their previous work level.

Prior to discharge the patient may be moved to a service department within the hospital. Again, these departments vary according to the facilities and cooperation of the hospital. Such departments commonly used involve working with portering, kitchen, laundry, gardening and hospital shop staff. Coping within a normal work environment, where patients are expected to function as a member of staff, is a realistic test as to whether they will cope with open employment or not. Most short-term patients cope with this situation. The drawbacks of such a system are:

a. Time: short-term patients are only in hospital for a brief period, therefore they may need to progress through the stages (on the ward, in the work unit and attached to a service department of the hospital) quickly in order to benefit fully.

b. Facilities: some resources may not be available, for example, the hospital may not have a clerical unit. Therefore, assessing and retraining in clerical skills may need to be done on an 'ad hoc' basis.

c. Co-operation from service departments to place patients with them: these departments only have limited places for patients and many of them will be filled by long-term patients as part of their rehabilitation programme.

Finally, pre-discharge, the occupational therapist may be involved in helping the patient to fill in job application forms, to offer advice and support before the job interview and to introduce or re-introduce the patient to the Job Centre.

If the occupational therapist and the rest of the treatment team have carefully decided that a patient's chances of getting a job are slim, then alternatives must be sought. The patient must initially be counselled about the realities of the situation and helped to adjust accordingly. The occupational therapist has an important role to play during this stage. She must make the patient aware of his other skills which he can use to help increase his low self-esteem. Such skills must be recognised by the patient, and the occupational therapist should indicate how they may be used when the patient is discharged.

Ways of utilising an individual's skills are legion—there are many ways in which patients can be made to feel more worthwhile as members of society.

The voluntary network can absorb many different types of people and skills, for example:

a. acting as driver for local hospital/old folk's club

b. being a hospital visitor

c. providing entertainment at local residential establishment

d. organising fund raising events
e. helping in the office/shop of a charity
f. making tea for old folk's day centre.

This list is endless and only requires the skills of the patient to be matched to an appropriate agency.

Using skills the patient has acquired, in hospital or previously, it may be possible to set up a small non-profit/profit making business, for example printing, making simple wooden toys, leather articles or other marketable products. It is important, however, not to maintain control over such enterprise unless it is genuinely intended to create a form of 'sheltered' employment.

It is important to introduce the patient to available community resources so that leisure time is more productively utilised, for example through sports centres, libraries, further education classes etc. Some individuals may be willing to take up new hobbies such as gardening, keeping pidgeons or creating soft-ware for microcomputers.

Not all patients will accept help in this area but many individuals only require some advice and guidance to find the area they are to be involved in. Occupational therapists can use discussion of leisure interests as part of the overall programme. Patients can discuss what they can do and what is available. Guest speakers could be invited to talk about the use of volunteers in various areas. The patients may be encouraged to build up an information file which would be available to others including, for example, the time of openings of local centres, the cost of entry and any reductions available for unemployed people. This could be added to as more information is gained. The occupational therapist could also introduce visits to the sports centre etc, as part of the programme, so that patients are acquainted with local facilities. This area is covered in more detail within Chapter 11.

Pre-discharge, the patient and the occupational therapist should have some plans as to how his leisure time is going to be utilised. Introductions to voluntary bodies etc. should be made if this is what the patient plans to do. If a person is engaged in activities which offer a feeling of self-worth then they may be less likely to need other forms of personal support.

ACTIVITIES OF DAILY LIVING

In order to survive one needs certain self-care skills. In order to be an acceptable member of society one needs further self-care skills. Many short-term patients do not have problems in the basic aspects of self-care, such as hygiene, toileting, etc, but often require help in the more complex skills of budgeting, domestic management etc. All short-term patients should be, where possible, assessed in this area to ascertain the level of their self-care skills. This assessment can be done in several ways:

1. By talking with and observing patients informally to establish what kind of domestic routine they have and if they feel they have problems in this area. Most short-term patients can articulate their problems and should be able to give a clear indication of where they lie.
2. By discussing with ward staff whether they have noticed any deficit areas in self-care.
3. By completing a formal domestic assessment. This may be required if it is difficult to ascertain from the patient or the patient's relatives how he functions at the domestic level.
4. By observing the patient in self-care/domestic situations which are a continuing part of the occupational therapy programme, i.e. baking groups/grooming groups, etc.
5. By completing a home visit with the patient to see how he copes in a familiar environment. This is often done before discharge but there is no reason why it cannot be used as an assessment procedure as long as the patient is able to cope with it in the early stages of illness.

Once this baseline has been established then this part of the programme can be planned. Some patients will require little help in this area—they may be competent household managers whose problems lie in other areas. However, self-care activities can still form part of their programme whereby they can achieve an increase in self-esteem and responsibility by helping other patients who have problems in this area. As long as this is done with care and sensitivity, patients acting in an advisory capacity to other patients can be very therapeutic for both parties.

In meeting the needs of the patients who do have problems in self-care/domestic activities the occupational therapist must be aware of the time factor. Many of these patients will only be in hospital for a short period of time, therefore, establish what activities are important to the patient and work in them. The learning of self-care/domestic activities should begin with something which the patient, rather than the therapist, considers important. Occupational therapists must be aware of the different backgrounds from which her patients come and not try to inflict her standards on them. Does it matter that it is common practice for some people to have a milk bottle on the table instead of a china cream jug?

The learning of activities of daily living should be taught on a one-to-one basis or in small groups depending on the patient's problems. Some difficulties are unique, therefore requiring individual attention; others are shared, therefore small groups are appropriate. There are advantages and disadvantages to both situations and the therapist must weigh up the considerations before deciding which is best. Often a lack of time demands that a patient, who could ideally benefit from individual treatment, is placed in a small group. Unfortunately, this is one of the realities of practising within limited resources; such constraints should not prevent the therapist from identifying and working towards the provision of a better service.

Often the problems patients have with activities of daily living are not in knowing how to carry out the activity for other reasons. A patient may well be able to cook a meal but does not do so because he does not like eating on his own and, therefore, would rather eat in a cafe even if this costs more than he can afford. This presents the occupational therapist with a different problem in that she must tackle the underlying reason and find some solution to it. She may encourage the patient to identify another person who lives alone and to get the patient to offer to cook for this person as well as for himself. This means that the patient has company at mealtimes; it may, of course, be difficult to arrange on a daily basis but, perhaps, could be done a few times a week.

Activities of Daily Living (ADL) groups such as beauty, baking, lunch and laundry groups have other benefits apart from the learning of self-care skills. They provide social opportunity in that people have to relate to each other, especially if there is limited kitchen equipment available. They help to increase self-esteem if people are complimented on their appearance or baking/cooking products following one of these sessions. They may help to increase social skills, where a patient has to act as hostess at a lunch group. Such a role includes inviting people to lunch, greeting them, serving the food, initiating conversation, etc. Often the informal relaxed atmosphere which can be produced during these groups make patients more willing to discuss their domestic problems and often a deeper discussion of other personal problems may follow.

There are a great many activities which could be considered under the heading of ADL. Broadly categorised they may include:
1. Personal hygiene
2. Cooking
3. Household cleaning
4. Laundry

5. Budgeting
6. Nutrition
7. Child care

As already mentioned not all patients will require help in all areas but general groups could be included in the programme which everyone could benefit from if only to retain skills which they possess in that area. The two most commonly used group are beauty/self-care and baking/cooking groups. Although these activities are typically seen as female-orientated, this need not be the case and many men enjoy and get a great deal of satisfaction from baking and cooking. Often, it opens up new horizons for them and some patients have gone on to attend evening classes in cookery.

Activities of Daily Living should be carried out in a unit which caters for the different activities. Facilities vary from hospital to hospital: in some places former staff living accommodation has been turned into teaching units with kitchen, bathroom, bedroom and living area. Other hospitals have purpose-built accommodation. Some hospitals have a lack of such facilities but many activities can be carried out on the ward. It is always preferable to complete a home visit with a patient who has been on an extensive ADL programme to see how they would cope at home in familiar surroundings. This often highlights problems which may not have been so apparent in hospital. Sensitivity must be shown when doing home visits; one middle-aged patient introduced her therapist to a neighbour, who had unexpectedly popped in, as her niece and explained her own absence as having been in hospital to get her corns done!

Some aspects of ADL can be carried out in practical and discussion groups. Budgeting and nutrition both lend themselves to this type of group where the menu is planned, shopped for and then cooked. Discussion can then follow as to the most economical types of food and how nutritious these are. Occupational therapists need to convey basic information about the value of the constituents of a normal diet. Sharing information about the difficulties of budgeting for a family can be beneficial and supportive to patients. Practical help can also be offered in conjunction with the social work/social services department. Rent, fuel bills, etc can be paid monthly and arrangements made for unpaid bills to be repaid gradually.

ADL activities may seem easy to the therapist but it is often a difficult area for patients to master and may take considerable time and practice before they become a part of the patient's life.

SOCIAL AND RECREATIONAL ACTIVITIES

Social and recreational activities cover an enormous range of possible activities which can be used with short-term patients. Because of their very nature most of the social and recreational activities which occupational therapists use are group orientated. The size of the group may vary but, as in any other group, dynamics will occur.

Social and recreational activities provide the fulfilment of many different needs, all of which contribute to a greater feeling of satisfaction and well-being on the part of the individual. Physical well-being can be developed or maintained. Many patients who are psychiatrically ill are in poor physical shape, any small exertion making them breathless, so social and recreational activities can improve this and leave them feeling physically more able to cope. Social interaction also occurs with social and recreational activities. Patients who are withdrawn have been known to participate during the more relaxed informal sessions. People relate to each other during these activities; they can practise socially acceptable behaviour within the context of the activity, i.e. waiting in turn, being a gracious loser, sticking to rules, etc. New social roles can also be tried out, for example, being leader which involves responsibility for the rest of the team, organising tournaments, etc. Cathartic release can also be achieved by some social and recreational activities; pent-up feelings can be released on a volleyball court or in wedging clay before making some pottery object. New hobbies can be identified and tried out which can be developed once the patient leaves hospital. This should help the patient to become more settled in the community and to meet new people if he attends clubs or classes associated with his hobby. Self-esteem is greatly enhanced by participating in social and recreational activities. A sense of achievement may be gained from participating in a group project which will help a children's home or a home for the elderly. Cognitive processes can be developed using social and recreational activities. Many patients suffer from conditions which affect their memory, concentration, attention-span, initiative, etc. Social and recreational activities can help the restitution of these processes by involving the patient in games or activities which gradually require more use of them. Such activities may include the playing of simple table games which require little attention, building up to more difficult games which require complex cognitive processes. Activities in which the patient has some interest should be used irrespective of the occupational therapist's personal tastes. Social and recreational activities also provide an opportunity for fun and enjoyment. Being a patient in a psychiatric hospital is often very difficult and may be associated with experiences of despondency and gloom. Allowing patients an opportunity to laugh can have a very potent therapeutic effect.

Maintaining contact with community resources is another aspect of social and recreational activities. Visiting the local swimming pool provides many things—dealing with traffic and people, using money, physical exercise, personal hygiene and the social skills involved in going for coffee afterwards. So social and recreational activities have many uses and form an important part of the occupational therapy programme.

To list all the social and recreational activities available would be lengthy and inconclusive so attention will be given to those more commonly found in short-term units. The facilities of the hospital and the surrounding area will of course affect the occupational therapy programme as will age, sex, diagnosis and social/intellectual background of the patients.

Games and sports may play a significant part. Team sports commonly used by occupational therapists are putting, football, cricket, volleyball, netball, basketball, skittles and rounders. Individual sports include billiards, table-tennis, darts, tennis, badminton, swimming. Different types of table games may also be included, such as dominoes, card games, beetle, bingo, scrabble, chess, chinese checkers or monopoly. Other types of games include charades, team games or others which overlap with those considered in conjunction with music, drama, movement and dance.

Hobbies can also be classified under a social and recreational heading. There are many hobbies which can be introduced or developed in the group setting; these include, for example, pottery, woodwork, metalwork, needlework, dressmaking, macrame, winemaking, photography and soft toymaking. Many of these activities can be continued outside the hospital when the patient is discharged. The occupational therapist may offer one session each week within which the patients can experiment with different types of hobbies. Quizzes and discussion groups can also be used. There are many different ways of organising quizzes, which may include the use of books, pictorial material and specialist topics. Discussion groups also can take many forms including balloon debates, current affairs or specific topics.

There are other miscellaneous social and recreational activities which do not fit into any defined category: yoga, keep-fit, all types of dancing, relaxation and art which are extensively used in occupational therapy programmes. Outings also form a large part of social and recreational activities. These can involve visits associated with sports, e.g. swimming pool, sports centre, trampoline centre, etc., or with some other interest—art gallery, museum, motor shop, special exhibitions, etc. It is more useful to the patients if they can decide where to go and be involved in the planning.

Group projects often play a part in occupational therapy programmes. The projects can be various but patients tend to be more motivated towards those which have a valid contribution to the needs of those who are deprived. Making toys for a local children's home or hospital often prompts patients who are very self-orientated to think of other people rather than of themselves. If a visit to the home to meet the children and staff can be organised this, again, increases motivation. Another group of people who are often identified as being deprived are elderly people; patients are often motivated to work together to produce something for the local old people's home. This can take the form of some fund-raising event, for example, a jumble sale or sponsored event.

There are patients who previously have only participated in social and recreational activities to a limited degree. These patients need to experience different types of activities so that they can identify those which they may like to explore further. The occupational therapist, in suggesting possible activities, must consider the facilities available in the community and the financial aspect of the activity. If the patient has limited financial resources it is unlikely that he will be able to be involved in activities which require a considerable financial outlay.

Units operating on a crisis intervention model require a different approach to constructive activities. Because of the relatively short period of time the patient is in hospital, the occupational therapist will probably only be able to assess the patients in terms of ADL, social, recreational and work skills. Her programme must, therefore, be carried out in the community either by herself or by a community occupational therapist. Working with psychiatric patients in the community is a new area for occupational therapists. There have been occupational therapists employed in the community for many years but the main bulk of their work involved dealing with physically disabled clients. Occupational therapists are beginning to meet this challenge and to use constructive activities within the community either in local day centres or in the clients' own homes. Obviously, these activities will require

218 OCCUPATIONAL THERAPY IN SHORT-TERM PSYCHIATRY

a degree of adaptation to fit into the lifestyle and facilities available to the client and will require the occupational therapist to use her ingenuity. This is a challenging area of occupational therapy opening up for the future.

Another factor occupational therapists often have to consider when using constructive activities is temporal adaptation. Here the occupational therapist must be concerned with the balance of time spent by patients on the various activities. Some satisfactory balance between ADL, work and leisure must be achieved. Some individuals do not have any balance between these three areas and may totally neglect one area. The occupational therapist must help these individuals to develop skills which would make it more balanced. The 'workaholic' who has no leisure pursuits will find retirement difficult and may suffer psychological stress; the housewife who was totally concerned with self-care, domestic and child rearing skills may suffer from problems of adaptation when her children leave home. Both these types of patients require help to re-adjust their lives to compensate for what they have lost and to gain satisfaction from new interests or skills which they have never developed.

Constructive activities are essentially a 'here and now', action-orientated process which involve learning through being involved in activity. Activities which are used are familiar, and realistic and specifically geared to individual needs. They are orientated round the three main areas of life—self-care, work and leisure. Patients are helped to develop new or more effective skills which will help them to cope with their present situation. Little emphasis is put on past events, more emphasis is placed on what is happening in the present and how the patient can be helped to cope with this.

BIBLIOGRAPHY

Briggs A K, Duncombe L W, Howe M L, Schwartberg S L 1979 Case simulation in psychosocial occupational therapy. F A Davies, Philadelphia
Cornes P 1982 Employment rehabilitation. Manpower Services Commission, London
Hughes P L, Mullins L 1981 Acute psychiatry care—an occupational therapy guide to exercise in daily living skills. Charles Slack, New Jersey
Mercer F 1981 Handbook of indoor social activities. P T M Press,
Mosey A C 1973 Activities therapy. Raven Press, New York
Mosey A C 1981 Occupational therapy. Raven Press, New York
Reed K, Sanderson S R 1980 Concepts of occupational therapy. Williams and Wilkins, Baltimore
Wansborough N, Cooper P 1980 Open employment after mental illness. Tavistock Publications, London
Hopkins H L, Smith H D 1978 Willard and Spackman's Occupational therapy, 5th ed. J B Lippincott Company, New York

11

Leisure

INTRODUCTION

A visitor to the occupational therapy department of a psychiatric hospital would observe people involved in a plethora of activities. The discerning visitor would see personal care programmes, domestic and social activities, social skills and cognitive training, craft and industrial work and programmes based on psychodynamic, behavioural or developmental theories. A glance through the department assessment forms would reveal records concerning hygiene and dressing and skills needed to run a home. Mobility would be assessed, particularly outside the home in the community in coping with crowds and various forms of transport. Information would be available on ability to relate to people, and on memory, orientation, concentration, numeracy and learning. Work skills would be recorded concerning relationships within the work situation, use of tools and time, and production of goods in terms of quality and quantity.

A brief appraisal of the activities to be seen and a quick review of the assessment forms available may lead the visitor to assume that the orientation within occupational therapy is towards the fundamental activities required to cope in a community as independently as possible. Emphasis appears to lie on taking care of personal needs, coping with basic domestic activities, relating to other people, being orientated in time, place and person, and earning a living through work. Such an assumption is, of course, correct.

The visitor, however, may comment on the scant, and in some cases non-existent, attention that is given to leisure activities. He may point out that up to five hours per day are available to a working person for leisure and that little concern is shown for what clients will do with their time when away from the hospital. He may also note that many activities used in occupational therapy, crafts and social activities in particular are considered to be leisure activities outside the therapeutic setting. He may mention that the therapist has given only passing recognition to their intrinsic leisure value but has chosen to use them purely for their therapeutic value as, for example, modes of expression or communication, or for their qualities which facilitate improvements in concentration, social skills or manual dexterity.

If such an omission becomes apparent, therapy programmes may be re-designed to include leisure rehabilitation in the occupational therapy curriculum.

The objective of this chapter is to facilitate such an inclusion through a brief analysis of leisure in a society, different types of leisure activities and problems which may occur regarding leisure for people suffering from mental illness. It will conclude with a discussion on how this knowledge can be applied to developing occupational therapy programmes in order to facilitate satisfying and productive use of leisure time for mentally ill clientèle.

AN ANALYSIS OF LEISURE

What is leisure?

There are three basic concepts associated with leisure: time, activity and state of mind (Godbey, 1980).

Leisure time is considered to be time available when one may choose activities without the obligations associated with work. It is the time which is not sold for economic gain but left over when all the necessities of life and work have been dealt with. It is commonly known as free time during which the participant exerts a degree of choice over his exertions.

Leisure is also associated with activity in that certain occupations or pastimes are considered to be separate from work and are indulged in for pleasure rather than production or economic remuneration. Such activities may be chosen for rest, such as sunbathing or watching television; for amusement such as visiting the theatre; or for expending emotional or physical energy in, for example, listening to music or playing sports. They may be chosen to improve education by attending night school classes; to be creative, through writing stories; or for making social contact with acquaintances, friends and relatives, by inviting people round to dinner, for example.

Leisure also connotes a pleasurable state of mind resulting in a feeling of freedom and well-being. The state of mind may be unhurried or tranquil or alternatively may be one of excitement, stimulation or creativity.

A workable definition therefore may be: leisure is time left over from work when a person involves himself in activity, or non-activity, of his own free will, for pleasure and not for remuneration, and enjoys a feeling of well-being, relaxation or stimulation.

Leisure, however, is not static phenomenon but changes in response to societal changes. A brief consideration of its changing nature is informative.

Historical development of leisure

Leisure patterns reflect the culture in which they exist, and change in response to changes in society. In hunter/gatherer and agrarian societies work and leisure merged and did not appear as well-defined separate entities (Cheek & Burch, 1976). Three to four hours of labour per day provided the necessities of life, and the relaxed pace allowed for the inclusion of leisure pursuits into work activities. There was time for social contact, for talking and laughing during work and many festivities such as harvest celebrations related to work.

Compare this to nineteenth century Britain at the height of the industrial revolution when the need for cheap labour was acute and work people laboured for sixty to seventy hours a week in noisy, overcrowded conditions which disallowed social interaction during work time. Also, there was little time, energy or money left over after work for leisure activities.

Conditions changed, however, and as a result of the developments in trade unions, education for working people, mechanisation and technology, accompanied by a reduction in the length of the working week and increases in wages, people had more free time, money and energy to devote to leisure activities. Gradually, leisure has developed separately from work and indeed for some has usurped work as a central life interest and has become more important than work.

One cannot discuss changes in work and leisure patterns without considering the Protestant work ethic (Weber, 1904). Max Weber links the development of the belief in hard work as a virtuous activity with Calvinism. A minority of chosen people were thought to be pre-ordained to reach a State of Grace in the eyes of God. This state could be displayed through diligent hard work and the resultant accumulation of material goods which were not spent or used for pleasure but were re-invested. Non-work pleasurable activities were discredited and Weber advocates that this ethos nurtured the development of capitalism and industrialisation in Britain and Europe. Capital industries were labour intensive, the demand for cheap labour was great, work was considered virtuous and leisure became very secondary. During the twentieth century leisure, as has already been discussed, has of course evolved in importance, but the Protestant work ethic is still strong and work still has a particular value in our society. This value is recognised by financial remuneration and status. Does not the Registrar General formalize the class system in his classification of occupations and, indeed, do not occupational therapists similarly pay allegiance to the work ethic by the emphasis placed on work activities? Is there not still stigma attached to unemployment?

One can, therefore, note the gradual change from a society where leisure and work were less distinguishable from each other to a society where work was predominant and leisure, except for the rich and aristocratic, was practically non-existent, to our present society where leisure and work are separate but still closely linked. This link is worthy of further discussion.

Leisure and work

Work and leisure style

Work affects both the time and energy available for leisure activities and also the leisure style an individual may adopt outside work.

Parker (1976) suggests that three models are apparent which illustrate the effect of work on leisure style.

1. *The extension model* suggests that people with personally satisfying jobs which allow a high degree of autonomy such as doctors or artists, are less likely to differentiate between work and leisure. Indeed work and leisure time activities will often merge. This model also suggests that these people will have more varied and satisfying out-of-work-time experiences.

2. *The opposition model*. Work is hard, sometimes dangerous, and often detrimental to the worker's well-being, for example, coal mining and heavy industrial work. Leisure activities tend to be totally separate from work, valued of far greater importance and often participatory in nature. Leisure provides compensation for hardships at work.

3. *The neutrality model*. Work is monotonous, boring and not particularly fulfilling, but neither is it oppressive, for example,

routine office work. Involvement at work tends to be passive and mundane. Leisure activities are not related to work nor are they opposed to it, but tent to be bland and demand more passive involvement.

Karl Marx similarly analysed the connection and stated that leisure patterns reflect work patterns. If man is alienated in his work he will also be alienated in his leisure. Developing a Marxist theme, C Wright Mills suggests that if people are manipulated to work as a mass labour force such as in mass production industries, they can also be manipulated to enjoy mass leisure such as spectator sports, TV watching and Bingo playing.

Work and leisure merged

The link between work and leisure can also be discussed in terms of the impingement of one upon the other. As in the old hunter/gatherer and agrarian societies, though not to the same extent, leisure activities can be included in work. Satisfying social interactions take place during tea, coffee and lunch breaks and friendships can be made in the work setting. Professional conferences can be held in pleasant locations and business can be done during lunch, dinner or a game of golf. Leisure activities may be formally provided by employing bodies; for example, industrial firms or local authorities may support social or sports centres or sponsor pleasurable events such as dances and sports tournaments.

Alternatively leisure activities can involve work, often of an arduous and unpleasant nature, which can lead to hardship and danger. Mountaineering can be wet, dangerous, lonely; skiing requires tremendous physical effort. People will often voluntarily involve themselves in tasks which they would not undertake as a paid occupation, such as cleaning out canals. Indeed, they will often pay to work under the guise of leisure, for example in conserving natural areas of beauty or interest, by joining schemes run by organisations such as the National Trust, to fell trees, mend fences and clear rural areas.

Leisure and industry

Yet another aspect of the work/leisure connection concerns the increase in the number of people who are earning their living in the burgeoning leisure industries which have grown rapidly to respond to demand and, indeed, have in their turn created demand. The Do-It-Yourself industry is rapidly expanding and the travel industry is well established. The caravan and camping trade provides mobile, portable holiday homes and pleasant, conveniently located sites in which to place them. Leisure centres abound and house expensive consumer sports equipment. A recent development is the health industry, which has produced a demand for special clothing, equipment and food.

The link between work and leisure is arguably strong but it is not indisputable. Roberts (1976) suggests that the link should be viewed with a degree of scepticism and that the concepts of leisure and work may be totally unconnected. Two obvious examples of the weaker link are the rich who have permanent voluntary leisure and the unemployed who have involuntary leisure thrust upon them.

Kaplan (1960) defines five different kinds of free time, some of which are, and some of which are not, associated with work:
1. Permanent voluntary leisure of the rich
2. Temporary involuntary leisure of the unemployed
3. Regular allocated voluntary leisure of the employed on holiday
4. Temporary incapacity of the employed, permanent incapacity of the disabled and voluntary retirement of the aged
5. Free time of the unemployed, elderly and disabled.

To summarise this particular discussion, leisure is a changing phenomenon which responds to societal changes including those in religion, the economy and technology, and is very much a product of a modern industrial society. The discussion will now shift from leisure and society to leisure and the individual and the meaning leisure has during different stages of the life cycle.

Leisure and the life cycle

The choice and function of leisure activities varies according to age and family circumstance (Parker, 1976).

Childhood

During childhood, leisure is usually associated with play, particularly for the pre-school child when time has not as yet been institutionally divided into obligatory school activities and non-obligatory activities.

The schoolchild's leisure time is more structured but still spent in play. During play a child expends energy, develops motor and social skills, phantasises and fulfils dreams, imitates and practises adults skills. Parker suggests that working class children exhibit more aggression and independence in play, are less protected and tend to sort out their own problems, whereas middle class children receive more parental protection, seek parental arbitration when problems arise and play in more formally defined and protected areas such as gardens.

Adolescence

During adolescence leisure becomes more colourful and varied and is influenced by peer group pressure or youth culture rather than by the family. Self-styling becomes apparent when the adolescent presents himself to the world in a chosen style of dress, behaviour or manner. Participation in sports activities and physical recreation is very evident.

Young adulthood

This is a period which begins very energetically, for men in particular, with a noticeable involvement in a variety of activities outside the home, including sports. Gradually, a more domestic orientation develops, when leisure activities become more home-centred. Women become less involved in physical recreation and become more interested in crafts, TV and hobbies. Men tend to continue their interest in physical recreation longer than women but they develop domestic interests such as Do-It-Yourself and gardening activities. Similarly, their TV viewing increases. A class differentiation is also apparent here, in that white collar workers tend to participate more in formal groups and organisations than blue collar workers. Single people, however, tend to continue their involvement in more varied leisure activities outside the home, men more than women.

Middle age

In middle age, domestic responsibility is usually reduced and more money becomes available for leisure activities outside the home. Men, in particular, may increase their participation in active leisure activities but, gradually, active participation tends to become more and more restricted. Ken Roberts (1970) suggests that this may be due not only to a possible decline in mental and physical vigour but also to the fact that much 'fun' industry is directed towards the young and people may experience social inhibition in joining in certain activities.

Elderly

Health and mobility of course become important factors in influencing leisure in later years. Activities take longer to do and participation in pastimes such as gardening, sport, crafts, walking and shopping declines. Parker reminds us that over 7000 social clubs exist in England and Wales especially for the elderly but less than 7 per cent of all the elderly will attend in one week. Cumming and Henry (1961) in their disengagement theory suggest that people may gradually withdraw and reduce social interaction and may indeed become increasingly pre-occupied with themselves, men more than women. Women are possibly less affected because their life style changes less in that their domestic responsibilities continue.

Leisure, then, has infinite variety. It can be considered in terms of time, activity and state of mind. It changes according to changes in society and is influenced by work, ethical beliefs, class and the life cycle and life style.

But now let a more pragmatic approach be adopted in the consideration of different types of leisure activities.

Types of leisure

Materially based leisure

This type of leisure has fostered and in turn has been fostered by the tremendous development in the leisure industry. Participation requires money. It may demand acquisition of tangible objects, such as cars, videos, records, sports equipment, clothes, second homes and caravans. It may involve visiting specially contrived leisure centres such as Safari Parks, Disney World, holiday camps, or participating in organised schedules such as cheap package holidays. Materially based leisure is allied to an industrial society and is the result of increased productivity. Access to this type of leisure activity depends primarily on having the money to pay for it.

Physical exercise

These leisure activities are often associated with physical fitness, concern for health or with an aesthetic sense of enjoyment derived from being outside. Included in this category are activities such as walking, climbing, bicycling, keep fit, swimming and jogging. Some activities require expensive specialised equipment such as mountaineering equipment but many, such as swimming and jogging, can be done with little financial outlay.

Eating and drinking

Within the home, activities include cooking for pleasure, now done by men and women, entertaining at home, and beer making. Outside the home, participants may eat out in restaurants, picnic or visit public houses.

Self styling

This is a concept discussed by Irving Goffman (1959). The term implies the application of a conscious effort in the presentation of oneself to the outside world through choice of such things as house style, clothes, make-up, jewellery, home decoration, choice of car and, indeed, choice of partner. Ideally, one presents oneself to the world in a way that is personally satisfying.

Crafts

Craft work is personally satisfying, labour intensive and needs relatively little financial outlay. Tools are re-usable. It may be done in the home or at Adult Education classes which are organised at special centres and provide instruction and necessary equipment. Craft activities can be both creative and utilitarian and include sewing, knitting, upholstery, painting, flower arranging, weaving, pottery, model making, dressmaking, to list a few of the more popular craft activities undertaken in the home or at Colleges of Further Education.

Mass entertainment

This tends to be 'other-directed' in that it is organised and presented to an audience and requires only passive involvement. Included in this category are spectator sports, Bingo, cinema attendance, listening to the radio and television viewing. Over 90 per cent of British households have a television and because of its well-established place in the British household it is worthwhile discussing this particular leisure activity in greater detail. Godbey (1980) discusses television viewing as a form of escapist behaviour which provides a sense of catharsis for a fatigued body and fatigued psyche in that television programmes are usually predictable, relatively pleasant, and involve little real choice or investment of self. It is a typical way of spending time as a family and can provide phantasy, education and passive social contact as well as entertainment.

Other forms of mass entertainment based on the communication media are book, magazine and newspaper reading, which reach a wide audience and are relatively inexpensive and can indeed be indulged in free-of-charge at the local library.

Family leisure

The discussion on television could be extended into this category, as television watching is a form of entertainment and killing time often undertaken by the family. In addition, parents and children as a unit are catered for by holiday industries such as holiday camps and package tour operators. Less expensive family leisure pursuits include swimming and sports activities, particularly in leisure centres, or visits to organised and supervised parklands such as public and national parks. Former adult domains such as public houses now provide family rooms where children are welcome. Home based family leisure pursuits include playing games, reading stories, model making and craft work. Religious institutions such as the churches, mosques and synagogues also provide a focus for social interaction within the family.

Educational leisure pursuits

Formal organisation of educational leisure pursuits is done by a number of educational institutions. Local Colleges of Further Education provide Adult Education through day and evening classes in a wide range of subjects, including technical skills, crafts and academic subjects to examination level. In addition, special groups may be catered for. Pre-retirement classes are organised for people approaching retirement age and classes may be run for people already retired, such as cookery sessions for the elderly which provide both social and practical functions. Special courses may also be organised for the mentally handicapped. Courses of a more instructional or academic nature are also run locally through the Open College scheme in which adults may attain or upgrade basic academic qualifications. Other educational courses can of course be run by organisations such as the Worker Educational Association (WEA) or by local special interest groups or religious institutions.

Home based educational leisure activities are provided by the mass media. Radio and television provides formal Open University courses which lead to nationally recognised qualifications as well as informative programmes of a general educational nature. The local library is of course another source of home educational pursuits.

Special interest leisure pursuits

Special interests are, of course, wide and varied. They can be primarily solitary occupations, such as stamp or coin collecting, or group activities, such as amateur dramatics or belonging to a rambling club. Most special interests, however, are catered for by clubs, societies, associations or organisations which offer expertise, support, a focal point, and if necessary specialised equipment to enthusiasts. Lists of special interest groups and their venue are obtainable through the local press, local library or information centre at the Town Hall.

Male–female leisure activities

The sharp differentiation between male and female leisure pursuits which existed a hundred years ago, when women's activities tended to be home-centred and men's activities centred outside the home, is less evident. Indeed, a conscious effort has been made within schools to educate all children in a variety of potential creative leisure activities. The difference between male and female leisure pursuits is slight in young and single people but tends to become distinct in married people, particularly those with children. Men tend to remain involved in physically active sports longer, while women tend to become more craft orientated. Both will share interests in Do-It-Yourself activities and watching television.

Entertainment

The term is used to imply activities which provide amusement or pleasant occupation, often by viewing a public performance of a play, opera or music. Such activities are provided in most towns by amateur operatic or dramatic groups and visiting or resident companies who offer performances to a public audience. Many groups or theatres will offer group concessions or reduced ticket prices to children, students, the elderly and the unemployed. Some cinemas, also, will provide reduced rates for select groups for weekday matinee performances or on special evenings during the week. Occasionally, performances require no entrance fee, for example church organ recitals and band concerts in the park.

LEISURE AND THE PSYCHIATRIC PATIENT

Let us now apply our considerations about leisure to the acute psychiatric patient. Our deliberations so far have focussed on a brief sociological survey of leisure in society and a practical analysis of different types of leisure, but now it is necessary to recognise the difficulties which may be encountered by a person suffering from mental illness. These difficulties may be discussed under three distinct headings: physical and material, social and psychological.

Physical and material problems

Many, though by no means all, the leisure activities already discussed require some financial outlay. One may need to purchase specialised items and equipment, pay membership or entrance fees, rent equipment or accommodation, or buy food or drink. These incurred costs are an obvious major problem to anyone whose income is limited, such as recipients of invalidity, unemployment or supplementary benefits.

A large number of leisure pursuits are indulged in away from the home; sports activities occur in the open and in leisure and sports centres; concerts and plays take place in centrally located special facilities; walking and sailing are usually done in the countryside; eating out is done in restaurants.

Similarly, many less ambitious pursuits, such as attendance at evening classes or speciality interest groups, are usually organised in some central location away from the home. Transport is, there-fore, necessary and if none is available the participant must organise, co-ordinate and pay for it, which again is difficult for someone living on a limited income or who has difficulty in using public or private transport.

Availability of leisure pursuits is also important. Availability varies from area to area, and from one local authority to another.

An interested person may be unable to participate in the activities of his choice simply because of lack of provision in the area in which he lives. For example, the urban resident in a densely populated, inner city, impoverished area will not have access to most sporting activities and the rural dweller will have limited access to adult education facilities.

Social problems

Many leisure activities involve interaction with other people, and this social contact can generate problems for mentally ill people if they get adverse reactions from the general public or if their social skills are poor.

Goffman (1963) discusses stigma as a societal reaction which emphasises specific personal attributes, which are evaluated negatively and considered as undesirable. These undesirable traits are remembered as the dominant feature of the stigmatised person and therefore 'spoil' his identity and categorise him as being deficient or deviant. Stigmatisation can and often does occur in people who suffer or who have suffered from mental illness. As a result they may experience several typical adverse reactions from people they meet both at work and socially. Some people may fear violence, unpredictability, or the occurrence of the florid signs of mental illness such as hallucinations or mania. Others may feel that responsibility for the person may fall upon them while others may misinterpret the symptoms of mental illness as unfriendliness, laziness or weakness of character. Consequently scapegoating, ridicule or avoidance may occur.

Inadequate social skills resulting from either pre-morbid or secondary handicaps can of course limit or impair social interaction and the person will experience difficulty in initiating, sustaining and controlling relationships with individuals or groups he may encounter in the pursuit of leisure. Potential hazards can occur even in seeking information about interests formally or informally in face-to-face contact, by telephone or through correspondence. Making initial contact, relating to strangers, or meeting individuals or a group again after discharge from hospital, is threatening, particularly if one's coping behaviour is limited. There is an additional difficulty which relates to stigma, in fielding possible impertinent, tactless or hurtful remarks made by acquaintances and friends.

Psychological problems

Primary handicaps associated with mental illness create tremendous problems with social relationships and can prevent the sufferer from partaking in or enjoying leisure pursuits as well as he may like to. Barriers may be obvious, such as interference from obsessive—compulsive rituals, hallucinations or delusions. They may result from misinterpretation caused by illusions or paranoia, or indeed barriers may be total due to extreme aniety or depression.

Other symptoms are equally problematic. A poor self-image makes stress control difficult and causes avoidance of situations which test ability or capability such as sailing, creative work and competitive sports. Inability to compete is in itself a problem in a competitive Western society and hinders comfortable involvement in most activities which involve spending time with other people, from quiet activities such as craft work in an evening class to energetic team games. Flatness of emotion makes social relationships difficult as well as reducing the thrill, exhilaration and pleasure that is possible from, for example, producing a satisfactory item of creative work, listening to a favourite piece of music, supporting a winning team at a football match, or engaging in strenuous or controlled physical activity. Low levels of frustration makes learning, coping with disappointment and waiting difficult, and inability to cope with change or the unknown causes stress and anxiety.

In addition, over-protection from either the family, who want to save their relative from exposure, stress or rebuttal, or from the caring institution, who fear relapse, may cause overdependence and reduce exposure to many pleasurable activities.

In consequence, a person suffering from mental illness may be attracted only to passive observer non-participant types of leisure activities which make little or no demands, such as television watching, walking in unthreatening places or housebound activities. Many may indeed avoid leisure activities altogether, preferring anonymity and non-involvement.

Several problems which have been discussed regarding leisure pursuits can occur, of course, regardless of the potential participant's state of mental health, but these problems can be compounded or concentrated if a person as a result of illness is unable to organise or problem solve in a way which he would like. Now let us discuss possible intervention strategies the occupational therapist may adopt in order to facilitate the pursuit of leisure activities for a person suffering from mental illness.

OCCUPATIONAL THERAPY

Leisure rehabilitation

The occupational therapist can and does use many of the leisure activities discussed as therapeutic media within the treatment programme in order to achieve formally desired goals in other areas of need such as social or work rehabilitation. This particular use of leisure activities is not the primary concern of this chapter, however. The emphasis in this context lies in the use of these activities as purely pleasurable pastimes that have a broader, less formally therapeutic value, as do similar activities for the well person. Consideration will be given to the occupational therapist's function in enabling a mentally ill person to participate in suitable leisure pastimes through a programme of leisure rehabilitation.

The occupational therapist

The occupational therapist as gatekeeper

The therapist is able to facilitate access to leisure activities by being a source of information through which an interested person may gain knowledge of suitable pursuits. She should be aware of and keep a resource file of what is available in the locality either through special interest groups, statutory or voluntary provision. She should be aware of any self-help or support groups such as Alcoholics Anonymous or MIND, which may organise social gatherings for mentally ill persons or their families, and also be cognisant of what Local Authority provision is available through the Recreation and Amenities and Education Departments.

The resource file would include information on leisure centre provision, sports activities and educational or hobby courses run by local Colleges of Further Education, including any courses for special groups such as mothers with young children, the elderly or persons prior to retirement. Some facilities will organise special arrangements to enable people to participate, for example a creche to allow young mothers to join keep-fit or swimming groups. Useful information would also include details of local library provision, local museums and exhibitions. The therapist should also provide access to information on services provided by special interest groups such as local dramatic or music societies, chess, rambling or stamp collecting clubs; by private enterprise such as theatres, cinemas, private sports clubs, and by national organisations such as the National Trust or National Society for the Protection of Birds.

Some knowledge of holiday provision which offers suitable organised holidays such as Holiday Fellowship may also be useful.

Information is available from the Local Authority such as Departments of Education or Recreation, Colleges of Further Education, Tourist Information Centres, Libraries and appropriate resources such as travel agents and central offices of national organisations. Such information could be made available in the course of leisure rehabilitation or through special Leisure Advisory Centres which are organised within the hospital.

The occupational therapist in habilitation

As well as providing information, the therapist can of course assist the mentally ill person to participate in leisure activities by facilitating development of the appropriate skills one needs to enjoy such activities. Fruitful participation in leisure pursuits requires cognitive and social skills which, because of pre-morbid or primary handicaps, may not be available to a sufferer of psychiatric illness. Through an appropriately planned occupational therapy programme which includes assessment and goal setting, such skills can be learned and practised through involvement in selected activities such as group work and social skills training.

The occupational therapist as teacher

As well as knowing what types of activities are available and acquiring appropriate cognitive and social skills, the participant also needs practical skills to enable him to enjoy his leisure time. The occupational therapist, within the resources available to her, is able to teach suitable skills and arrange practise situations within the department. Within her teaching repertoire are craft activities, painting, drawing, appreciation of books, poems and music, dancing, general social activities, some sports activities such as bowls or tennis, discussions, appreciation and evaluation of the mass media, cooking, wine or beer making, gardening, dressmaking, woodwork and metal work. In addition, the therapist can arrange learning experiences in the community through visits to the theatre, museums, cinema, parks and riding schools. If activities are selected which are not within her repertoire or if knowledge is pursued beyond her teaching range, then she will be able to consult the resource file and make contact with appropriate people who can teach what she cannot.

The occupational therapist as supporter

The degree of support required for the participant
comfortable and proficient in practical or social leisure sk
Initially, structured maximum support can be given by the   ..apist
in accompanying the participant to venues outside the hospital.
Through continuous assessment and goal planning, support will be
modified and reduced. Throughout leisure rehabilitation the
programme should include discussion and goal setting prior to
participation, and analysis of experience afterwards. Support can
also be given within a patient group, and arrangement of appropriate group sessions is part of the therapist's supportive remit. In
addition, she will liaise with the participant's family or close friends
and offer advice and support to them by informing them of developments in the leisure rehabilitation programme and answering any
queries they may have. Her therapeutic approach will allow her to
determine and modify the amount and nature of the support
required.

The occupational therapist as provider

The discussion has centred on facilitating access to leisure pursuits
in the outside community, but for some people such involvement
will be temporary or permanently too threatening, and invoke an
unacceptable degree of stress. For those the occupational therapist
will become a leisure pursuits organiser and provider. Such provision is available in some locations in the formal social clubs run
for persons with more chronic illnesses. These facilities can also be
of positive use, possibly of a temporary nature, to the acutely ill
person where he can enjoy leisure activities in a sheltered environment and participate in social events, outings and special interest
groups which have been tailored to suit his needs.

An informed approach

Organisation of the leisure rehabilitation programme is, of course,
improved by an informed approach. The therapist will combine
knowledge of leisure with therapeutic skills to plan and implement
an appropriate schedule. A problem solving approach using the
occupational therapy process (Trombley & Scott, 1977; Willard &
Spackman, 1978) is an appropriate structure to use in organising
the therapeutic programme.

Assessment of the following areas is advocated:

1. The client's present interest in and ability to cope with leisure activities

This information will provide a baseline from which the client and therapist will work. As leisure is concerned with free will and pleasure, the client has to be totally involved in the programme planning, otherwise the process becomes anachronistic. It is he, in consultation with the therapist, who will decide at which point and to what extent leisure rehabilitation will be included in his therapy programme. Once included, the therapist will use her skills in planning and application to regulate direction and pace. Short-term goals will be formulated from this information.

2. The client's leisure interests and level of participation prior to onset of illness

This information will be obtained from the client himself, his family or any other relevant person. Such information is obviously subjective but is no less valuable as it will indicate the existence of pre-morbid handicaps, loss of function due to illness and previous lack of opportunity to partake in leisure pursuits. It will indicate whether rehabilitation or habilitation is necessary. If the client's leisure was previously satisfying then a rehabilitation approach will be adopted to prevent further loss of function and ease his re-involvement in normal life pursuits during and after recovery. If the client's leisure involvement was unsatisfactory to him or if, after discussion with the therapist, he wishes to improve his leisure interests, then a habilitation programme can be negotiated. Short-term and long-term goals will be formulated from this information.

3. Barriers to successful outcome

The therapist must analyse and define any physical, material, social or psychological barriers which impede success or which will cause modifications to the programme. Stress-related illness, for example, will produce symptoms such as anxiety which will interfere with enjoyment of leisure pursuits. The client's stress will also dictate that any programme should be carefully designed and monitored to control stress and that any leisure activities will produce a feeling of well-being and not anxiety.

4. The client's social status

Consideration of age, sex, class, occupation, marital state and social roles within the family, work and the community will allow a more informed and sensitive approach, both to suggesting suitable activities to a client and in turn to understanding his choice of pastimes. However, one obviously cannot be deterministic about these choices.

5. The client's environment

This will include assessment of both his immediate environment, such as family support and personal private space within the home, and the wider community environment, and what is available there in terms of possible leisure pursuits, their accessibility and cost.

6. The client's employment status

The link between work and leisure is historically strong, and problems in leisure rehabilitation are compounded if the client is unemployed. The functions of leisure will be increased. As well as providing pleasurable, freely chosen activities, leisure must also provide for time-killing, energy expenditure and self-esteem that an employed person will get from working. Leisure will provide similar functions for the retired worker also, but the retired will not suffer the same stigma as the unemployed.

Following assessment, problems and strengths can be defined. Problems will include pre-morbid handicaps, social, psychological and psychiatric problems associated with mental illness, limited income, poor social support, limited availability of leisure activities within the client's environment, and poor access to any that are available. Strengths will be in the client's proclivity for particular activities, any intellectual or physical assets he may have, appropriate family interest, ability to use public or private transport, adequate finance and availability of appropriate activities in the home or community environment. Long-term and, more immediately, short-term goals can be negotiated and defined by the client and the therapist.

Treatment planning and implementation will include exploration of possibilities, experimentation with different pastimes, learning new skills, role play, modelling, practice and real life experience, discussion and analysis. As has already been indicated there are many different types of activities to choose from. At the passive end of the scale is television viewing, which can be of tremendous value to someone under mental stress by facilitating relaxation, catharsis and reduction in social isolation. At the other end of the scale are active physical sports such as running, swimming or squash playing, which have the same effect in reducing mental stress, but also have the added bonus of producing physical well-being.

The choice of activities and the client's response need to be continually re-assessed by both the client and the therapist and long- and short-term goals modified as necessary.

In conclusion, the occupational therapist can combine her therapeutic skills with an informed approach to facilitate participation in appropriate leisure pursuits for the client suffering from mental illness. Inclusion of leisure rehabilitation programmes in the occupational therapy curriculum is of much value as the inclusion of work rehabilitation programmes; indeed, for some, such as the unemployed or retired, it is of more value as leisure becomes a work substitute. It is hoped that this chapter will ease the development of leisure rehabilitation programmes in departments where they have not previously existed.

SUMMARY

This chapter has defined leisure in terms of activity, time and state of mind. The link between society and leisure had been established and examples of concommitant changes in culture and leisure were given. Changes in leisure interests during the life cycle have also been discussed. Different types of leisure activities were analysed as were the specific problems which people suffering from mental illness may experience in pursuing non-work activities. The chapter advocates that the occupational therapist, combining her therapeutic skills with an informed approach, can facilitate leisure rehabilitation for mentally ill clients and that leisure rehabilitation should be an integral part of the occupational therapy curriculum.

REFERENCES

Bottomore T B, Rubel M (eds) 1963. Karl Marx: selected writing in sociology and social philosophy. Penguin Books, Harmondsworth

Burns T 1973 Leisure in industrial society. In: Smith M, Parker S, Smith C (eds) Leisure in society in Britain. Allen Lane, London

Cheek N H Jr, Burch W Jr 1976 The social organisation of leisure in human society. Harper and Row, New York

Cumming E, Henry W E 1961 Growing old—the process of disengagement. Basic Books, New York

Godbey G 1981 Leisure in your life. Saunders College Publishing, Philadelphia

Goffman E 1959 The presentation of self in every day life. Penguin Books, Harmondsworth

Goffman E 1963 Stigma: notes on the management of spoiled identity. Prentice Hall, New York

Haralambos M 1980 Sociological themes and perspectives. University Tutorial Press

Kaplan M 1960 Leisure in America. John Wiley and Sons, New York

Mills C W 1956 The power elite. Oxford University Press, New York

Parker S 1972 The future of work and leisure. Pratger, New York

Parker S 1976 The sociology of leisure. George Allen and Unwin Ltd, London

Roberts K 1970 Leisure. Longmans, Harlow

Roberts K, Clark S C, Cook F G, Semeonoff E 1976 On the relationship between work and leisure, A sceptical note. University of Liverpool Department of Sociology

Trombly A T, Scott A D 1977 Occupational therapy for physical dysfunction. Williams and Wilkins, Baltimore

Hopkins H L, Smith H D 1978 Willard and Spackman's Occupational therapy. J B Lippincott, New York

Strategic skills

INTRODUCTION

The work of an occupational therapist is not restricted to time spent with the defined patient: a large part of the day is spent working with colleagues. This time includes departmental meetings, meetings with other members of the treatment team, case conferences and other events. The role of the individual includes relating to others who are more senior and also to those for whom one is responsible. This latter group may include helpers who may have many years of experience but little formal training and also students from different disciplines.

Whilst the phenomenology in inter- and intra-professional relationships is usually only latent, it seems useful, nevertheless, to identify a few frameworks and strategic skills to ensure perfect satisfaction from such interactions. The material in this chapter goes only part of the way to attaining this goal, lack of space restricting academic discussion of the issues involved. Much of what follows will be familiar and may ring certain bells in the reader who recognises past experiences and rules of thumb. I hope that the experience of seeing it set out on paper by someone else will be of interest and use. This is, therefore, a practical guide to the conduct of meetings, negotiations, decision making and the exertion of influence.

MEETINGS

A surprising proportion of working time is spent in meetings. Meetings come in all shapes and sizes and for a wide variety of purposes. A characteristic of most meeting is that the participants resent being there and do not feel that the meeting meets their goals and needs. However, meetings are crucial in the coordination and planning of work and 'Meetings skills' are a legitimate professional acquisition for the occupational therapist.

It is useful to ask what is the actual purpose of each meeting—is it to collect information, to disseminate information, to plan projects, to provide support, to make decisions or to allow people to sound off? Is the meeting structured in such a way that these goals can be achieved? Are the necessary people present? Are there people present whose time is being wasted? It is really the chairman's duty to organise and structure the meeting, to ensure that the appropriate people are present for the relevant periods, and also to attend to the process of the meeting and keep it healthy and alive. It is, however, important that each and every member is clear about their role and duties, and how to use the meeting, if they are to acheive whatever it is that justifies them spending their time at the meeting.

Meetings as group events

Meetings are special group events in which there is often too little time to properly attend to the inevitable group process. The following frameworks are succint enough to be used in the busiest of meetings.

A psychologist, William Shutz, suggests that groups can be said to develop through three main processes.

1. *Inclusion*. A cluster of people congregate together and, whilst on the surface they will be discussing all sorts of things, the underlying theme is 'Do I belong? Do I want to belong? Do I want to belong if Sue Smith is involved?'. After a while and a certain amount of coming and going, an understanding about membership develops and the group can be said to have worked through its inclusion to establish a tentative—and fragile—boundary around it.

2. *Control*. The next theme is one of negotiating the norms and allegiances (amongst birds only is this the 'pecking order'). Members seek to check out the rules of the group such as how deeply will certain matters be discussed. This is done by almost invisible giving and denying of approval to comments that are too deep or too superficial for the comfort of the others. Meanwhile, members are checking out where they stand with other members and trying to find out how far they can depend on different people—and whom they are prepared to support. After a while the group may reach an implicit agreement over the rules and allegiances and can be said to have established a first and tentative degree of trust through working through the control theme. The group

then moves onto the third stage in which people know where they stand in this group and can get on with the work in hand, rather than feeling obliged to be sorting out their own personal relationships. This third stage is known as:

3. *Affect*. Feeling included and trustful, people can express and use their feelings, in a constructive and almost selfless way. The reader will be familiar with the working through of inclusion at many an event; control themes are most blatantly illustrated by the way in which a group of children start acting up and causing trouble just at the point when you thought that they were starting to get together. 'Control' can also be detected in the game playing, teasing or 'horseplay' or general testing out that goes on in groups of adults. When the membership of a group—or meeting—changes, the inclusion will be re-negotiated and the modified patterns of allegiance and possible shifts in norms have to be checked through before the group can return to working at the 'affect' stage. The cycle is also repeated if a group stays together for a while and the members want to make the intensity of involvement greater. For instance, a group of lads may have formed a functioning group in which to spend their evenings but one day one of them says that he is short of money so how about they all go and rob the Post Office. At this point some of the lads may want to step out of group (and maybe other lads join in) as the inclusion is re-negotiated. Then the group will turn to the control issues and negotiate the new norms—will they use violence? Will they not betray their friends if caught? They will also check out their allegiances to make sure that they can trust each other in the group. (About 30 per cent of solved crime is solved because someone 'grasses'.)

In a meeting it is important that everyone experiences a welcome and a gesture of inclusion—especially when it is likely that they do not really wish to be there at all. It is also necessary to permit a few minutes for the control themes to be worked through in a covert fashion so that people feel that they have made their gesture and established their presence. This may take only five minutes before the business can get started but if it is ignored then these personal issues will be being worked through at the expense of, and under the cover of, the item being discussed: the outcome of the case conference becomes less to do with the patient's condition and more to do with the score in the game of 'get the nurse/consultant/OT/etc.'

Shutz's framework is a quick way of working out where a group has reached. A second framework serves as a guide to what one can then do about it.

Table 12.1 The needs and functions of a working group

Task needs of the group i.e. for a clear goal for agreement about goal for plan of action and so on.	Must be met through task behaviour	Initiating Informing Clarifying Summarizing Consensus	IF these are performed adequately
Maintenance needs of the group i.e. for mutual support for clarity for mutual understanding and so on	Must be met through maintenance behaviour	Harmonising Gate keeping Encouraging Compromising Giving feedback	AND these are performed adequately
Individual needs of the members i.e. to belong to be respected for status for power for dependency and so on	Must be met through group task and maintenance behaviour. The residue manifests as personal or self-oriented behaviour.	Aggressive behaviour Blocking Dominating Avoiding Abandoning	AND individual needs are met in the maintenance behaviour of the group.

THEN you have a good group!

Task and maintenance

It is possible to consider behaviour in groups under the heading of either task behaviour or maintenance behaviour. Task behaviour is conduct which furthers the (defined) work of the group. Maintenance behaviour, on the other hand, is conduct that helps the group function productively. The model is derived from industrial production where, for instance, we are concerned with a drilling machine: task behaviour is drilling holes whilst maintenance behaviour is stripping it down, oiling it and so on. The optimum balance is where the maintenance behaviour is sufficient but not in excess of what is necessary to permit the task to be achieved. Too much task focus and, although a lot of holes will be drilled in the short term, the machine burns out: too much maintenance behaviour and few holes are drilled even though a year later the machine is still immaculate.

Groups in which there is insufficient maintenance behaviour may achieve a great deal in the short term but they, too, burn out in the medium term. Groups in which there is insufficient task behaviour become cosy but boring and ineffective. Group members need to be attentive to the balance of task and maintenance behaviour for otherwise the members will soon cease to get much satisfaction out of their membership.

Individuals have certain needs and requirements which are partially satisfied within a group. If the group is, in fact, a meeting then these needs are to both achieve the goals of the meeting and also to fulfil simple personal needs such as occur in any social situation. If these needs are not being met, then the individual is very likely to give up on the group meeting. We can schematise this pattern in 12.1. In order that the group or meeting should be able to achieve its goals and to work well, the task and maintenance needs of the group must be met and, through the satisfaction of doing this, the individual needs of the members must be met. Table 12.1 illustrates how each and every person in a group can lead that group towards the attainment of its goals.

This table is amplified below with examples of how the different types of behaviour may be recognised.

Two popular misconceptions are revealed by looking at the work of a group in this way. The first is that ordinary members are helpless when, in fact, a great deal can be done by asking yourself 'what is missing?' and, having identified it, making a contribution that will meet this lapse. This might be getting the group to move its

Table 12.2

Group task behaviour	Conduct that furthers the work of the group
1. Initiating	Proposes aims, ideas, action or procedures.
2. Informing	Asks for or offers facts, ideas, feelings, or options.
3. Clarifying	Illuminates or builds upon ideas or suggestions.
4. Summarising	Pulls data together, so group may consider where it is.
5. Consensus	Explores whether group may be nearing a decision; prevents premature decision-making.

Group maintenance behaviour	Conduct that helps the group function productively
1. Harmonising	Reconciles disagreements, relieves tension, helps people explore differences.
2. Gate keeping	Brings others in, suggests facilitating procedures, keeps communication channels open.
3. Encouraging	Is warm and responsive; indicates with words or facial expression that the contributions of others are accepted.
4. Compromising	Modifies own positions so that group may move ahead; admits error.
5. Giving feedback	Tells others, in helpful ways, how their behaviour is received.

Personal or self-orientated behaviour	Conduct that interferes with the work of the group
1. Aggressive behaviour	Attacks, deflates, uses sarcasm.
2. Blocking	Resists beyond reason, uses 'hidden agenda' items which prevent group movement.
3. Dominating	Interrupts, asserts authority, over-participates to point of interfering with others' participation.
4. Avoiding	Prevents group from facing controversy; stays off subject to avoid commitment.
5. Abandoning	Makes an obvious display of lack of involvement.

discussion on by doing a bit of 'clarifying' or 'summarising'; or it could be that a bit of 'gate keeping' is needed in order to bring in the shy but knowledgable person at the end of the table. This is a very powerful tool!

The second popular misconception is that if someone is behaving negatively in ways described under 'self-orientated behaviour' it is their fault. If someone (maybe you) is starting to 'dominate' or 'abandon' then you know that something is wrong with the group process that they are not getting sufficient satisfaction out of being involved in the work and maintenance of the group. It is, of course, possible that they are feeling tired or distracted, but on the whole there is no excuse for a meeting to be boring or unsatisfying to an essential member. Self-orientated behaviour is a symptom that the process is lacking and the balance between task and maintenance needs to be restored. It is too simple and entirely unproductive to make a personal attribution to the acting-out member. The truth of this is particularly evident when it is you who is acting out the self-orientated symptom!

There is of course a great deal more to be said about groups but in this practical pot-pourri we now turn to 'problem solving'.

Meetings and problem solving

In systems theory a problem is defined as 'the inappropriate solution imposed upon a difficulty'. I feel depressed—this is my difficulty in living (let's say its simple reactive to the break-up of my marriage)—so I drink: my drinking is 'the problem'. Problems in organisations are often the consequence of having to work with other people.

'Problem solving' is used here as a label to describe strategic planned thinking. Professional supervision is an example of structured thinking around a situation that needs understanding and some action or decision to be made. The structure offered here is in seven steps, (Social skills in Chapter 7 described a similar approach in a different way.)

1. Collect the information—not just through collating anecdotes but in an organised way.
2. Make sense of the information by referring to past examples, theories, conceptual models and so on, so that an understanding of the situation is created.
3. Identify at least three different strategies by which to meet this situation.
4. Choose one of them.
5. Identify how you will monitor the effectiveness of the ensuing action for later reference.
6. ACT!
7. Assess the outcome.

In supervision there is a great pressure to go straight from (1) to (4) to (6). Stages (2) and (3) are needed to step out of habitual panic responses!

There are two basic approaches towards problem solving, one based on analytic thinking and the other on intuitive feeling. Both are best in their appropriate circumstances. The analytic approach is most useful when the information is available, for example when one is working out what is the best way to travel to Aberdeen: the fares and timetables for coach, train and plane are available and the fares can be compared with travelling by car. Sometimes the information is not available—or is only available as one starts on the action. When preparing for an interview with a moody and erratic superior (or parent, or spouse), it is necessary to recognise that the careful preparation of what you will say will probably be ineffective, and will probably be entirely inappropriate. Under these circumstances the intuitive approach will be more effective, even if it is more anxiety provoking. Most people have had at least one experience of having rehearsed an interview to the extent that they are locked into that script regardless of the changed situation!

There is a wide variety of different models for problem solving. Most of them are different ways of making lists. (A friend of mine says 'beat entropy, make lists!) The interested reader can find a selection of these in an excellent book entitled 'The Manager's Guide to Self-Development' by Pedler and Burgoyne.

For an individual, when the problem solving is complete, the decision usually follows directly. In a meeting it is more complicated.

There are four main advantages to problem solving in a group:
1. It engages you in a more detailed interaction with the problem.
2. The different people can pool their different knowledge and information.
3. Errors get averaged out—and because of this people are more willing to use their imagination, secure in the knowledge that others will be limiting any possible eccentric consequences.
4. In the security and creativity of (3) it is more likely that someone will have a 'eureka' experience of genius which will get shared around.

The disadvantages of problem solving in a group is the time it takes—and that it is subject to the phenomenology of groups (see above) so well alluded to in the comment that a camel is a horse designed by a committee.

Meetings and decision making

Problem solving is at the heart of a great deal of the information processing that a meeting tackles but it is only the prelude to 'decision making'.

Problem solving is about the quality of the eventual decision but decision making is concerned with the structure which determines the likelihood that the solution or decision will be implemented. Even the best of plans come to naught if those who have to carry them out are not committed to them.

Imagine the principal administrator and his team have to decide between two plans, plan A and Plan B. The principal favours Plan A and, like everyone else; he knows that the plan he favours is the best one: he gives it a score of 100. His team favour plan B but, whilst they of course give Plan B 100, the principal 'knows' that it is no more than adequate as a plan and he only gives it 70. However, the principal recognises that if he imposes Plan A (which is best) on the team they will only be 50 per cent committed to implementing it and as a result, good though it is, in practice it will yield only 50 per cent of 100 Application Points. He also recognises that they would be 90 per cent committed to implementing Plan B (which he knows is inferior) but that 90 per cent of 70 is 63 Application Points.

Table 12.3

	Plan A	Plan B
Rated by Principal	100	70
Committment to implement	50%	90%
Application Points	50	63

Of course, the team who thought Plan B worth 100 see the Application Score as 90 but the principal is only concerned with his own criteria which, he sees, are better fulfilled by selecting Plan B. If the figures were different, then it might be better to insist on Plan A. Table 12.3 is just an example of the sorts of question that need to be asked when working in a team or an organisation.

In decision making, then, it is not sufficient to arrive at the correct solution to the situation but also to identify how to have that decision put into practice. This issue of commitment is crucial when we consider the nature of the work of the occupational therapist. There are many different structures in which decisions are made within an organisation but the list below describes just eight of the more common structures. All things being equal, the structure and way in which a decision is made will determine the degree of involvement, responsibility and commitment to that decision by the people involved (or left out).

1. *Consensus.* Technically—and this is how we use it—this means

that everyone involved supports the decision. Under the consensus structure, the decision is not ratified until everyone states their support for it.

2. *Agreement*. The decision made by agreement is one in which no-one disagrees—there may be abstentions but no voice is raised against the decision. This is sometimes known as 'nem. con.' in, for instance, the Co-operative Movement.

3. *Majority*. The decision is made when 51 per cent of those involved support it. The constitution of an organisation, for instance, a trade union, will stipulate what sort of majority is necessary for certain sorts of decisions; the decision to strike often requires a two-thirds majority and to change the constitution may require a three-quarters majority. The two party electoral system works on the 51 per cent majority—but more of that later.

4. *Minority*. This is where the decision is made by a subgroup (management group, working party, sub-committee etc.) of the decision-making body and on their behalf. This might be the executive and council of the professional body to whom will be entrusted the power to make certain decisions.

5. *Expert*. Where the decision is deferred and referred to the expert, then the group has used the 'expert structure' to make their decision. An example of this would be asking the hospital administrative staff to allocate car parking spaces since they (presumably) are in a better position to have picked up the appropriate skills and knowledge in this area (i.e. the best places go to those who have to use their cars most frequently).

6. *Averaging*. This is where a decision is made on the basis of the replies from a questionnaire by a sort of numerical averaging. This type of decision making by averaging also occurs when a paper is circulated and you are asked for comments in the margin. The British electoral system actually works in this way when there are three or more candidates and where the elected candidate may well have only collected 34 per cent of the votes cast.

7. *Authority with consultation*. The principal makes the decision but he asks his colleagues for their opinions first. The staff may say all sorts of things and he listens but then *makes up his own mind*. It is important that the principal is not coy, talking about wanting a 'quick consensus'.

8. *Authority without consultation*. Here the principal makes up his mind, makes the decision and only later—if at all—tells the other people what was decided on their behalf. Minor day-to-day

decisions are made under this structure: one hopes that the decision that these decisions may be made this way was made by a more discursive structure.

May I invite the reader to now re-read this section and check that these distinctions between each structure is clear. Think of your own examples for each one.

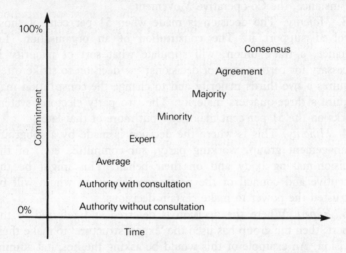

Fig. 12.1 Methods of decision making related to time and commitment.

Speaking personally, I expect all of my staff to be 100 per cent committed to what I decide on their behalf. Bitter experience has shown me that this is insane and unrealistic: I must recognise that those decisions which require commitment also require that I allow time for the appropriate structure—and recognise that if there is not enough support, for a decision that requires support, then the project is not viable. Similarly, it allows me to recognise those decisions which do not merit or need much time being spent on them—in this way I save the time to use it where it is needed. A colleague recently took over a very old-fashioned Elderly Person's Home: some changes were easy and immediate—such as no longer waking all residents at 6 a.m. Other decisions, in particular the instigation of a key-worker system, took over a year to accomplish since the final decision needed the commitment that is only created by using a majority/agreement structure.

An understanding of the relationship between the decision making structure and the commitment/time balance enables one to plan a schedule of work—and to encourage others to do the same.

It becomes clear that the meeting is not just pivotal in decision-making information processing, but that the way in which the meeting is organised, and set in the context of the rest of the member's work, determines how their work is helped or hindered by the individual and pattern of meetings. Before we turn to the precise duties of the chairman, let us remember the other ways in which business is transacted between members of an organisation. These include the infamous 'memo', the interview with one other person, the circulation of a discussion paper (it is much easier to read a paper than to hear someone talk their way through the same material—look at the way that lecturers arrange their lectures to amplify and discuss material already read—imagine how tedious it would be if they just read out of a book to the students!)

Some organisations get stuck into the habit of long meetings which seek to do too much and consequentially achieve very little. Imagine instead a meeting that is organised so that there is:

1. A brief period to catch up on any memos, reports and other bits of information best read immediately preceding the meeting.
2. Quarter of an hour for pairs or threes of people to quickly discuss matters that concern them only and would be tedious if discussed with the rest of the meeting as an uninvolved audience.
3. The meeting proper now starts with everyone prepared, with peripheral business complete and with members knowing that their participation will be relevant and appreciated.
4. If there is a lot of business, or if it separates into very different themes—such as administration and case discussion—then two

Table 12.4 Matching the type of decision to its appropriate level

Types of issue	Arenas or forums for the processing of information or decisions						
	Admin Officer	Snr Staff Meeting	Memo	Notice Board	Supervision Session	Staff Meeting	Etc
Case							
Discussion							
Staffing							
Policy Papers							
Resources							
Equipment							
Rotas							
Liaison							
Support							
Etc							
Etc							

short meetings are arranged rather than let one impossibly demanding session be imposed upon those present.

Table 12.4 shows a structure upon which it is possible to plan decision making, general information sharing etc. and the restriction of the agenda of meetings to what is practical, necessary and viable. Try filling it in to deal with your own situation. Order the sequence of 'forums' in order (1, 2, 3) for the processing of each type of issue.

Chairing a meeting

The role of the chairman is crucial in a meeting. It is alarming how many people have to chair meetings who have never had the opportunity to study or learn how to do it. Some people have been lucky enough to experience good chairing from others and have learnt ways of doing it from the models provided. Other people have not had such good luck and have had rather poor models to emulate. The notes below are based on an anonymous handout I found some years ago. I am very grateful to the author and I hope that he or she would approve of the alternations and additions I have made to it over the last couple of years. You will recognise some of the concepts already described in the first part of this chapter.

It is often said that meetings comprise a bunch of the unfit, appointed by the unwilling, to do the unnecessary. However, they are an intrinsic part of the work so it is necessary to make them as constructive as possible.

For the purposes of clarity and brevity this is written to emphasise the role of the chairman before, during and after meetings. This is not meant to imply that what is contained in the notes can be disregarded by those not occupying such positions. The other members need to know their roles and the process as well!

A meeting is a group and the chairman must steer the members through the inclusion stage (to create a sense of membership) and the control stage (negotiating allegiances and norms) if the discussion is to be productive. Without this, the people meeting may be more involved in working through their personal feelings and relationships than comprehending and working on the content of the meeting.

Responsibilities of a chairman

a. He must earn respect
b. He must respect the views of others

c. He must control
d. He must coordinate
e. He must distinguish between opinion and fact
f. He must lead
g. He must ensure progress is recorded.

A chairman, having accepted the role, must accept responsibility not only for the meeting but for what precedes and follows it.

Preceding

The chairman must ensure that the meeting has:

a. A purpose—because this sounds obvious it is often neglected. If you haven't got a purpose you do not need a meeting.
b. A secretary—provides good training for managers. Friendliness is important.
c. A minute-taker—the job can be circulated. It is not a popular job but it does provide valuable training.
d. An agenda—this should be as short as possible. It is better to cover a few subjects well rather than many badly.
e. A date and time—if a series of meetings are planned endeavour to fix each on a recognisable day, e.g. first thursday of every month. Allow time prior to the meeting for up-to-date information to be gathered.
f. A venue (location, accommodation, feeding)—consider the facilities required and the suitability of the room.
g. Essential fittings (chairs, tables, ashtrays, paper, ventilation, etc.)
h. Discussion openers and closers—prime people for these.
i. Follow-up arrangements—action to be taken, reporting back etc.
j. Winding up arrangements—seeing people off the premises, saying goodbye etc.

At the meeting

The agenda

The most important piece of paper at a meeting is the agenda. Like the tip of an iceberg it represents the visible portion of a large amount of otherwise unseen activity. The agenda embodies the plan of campaign which enables those responsible to achieve the objectives of the meeting. Hence, the agenda must be seen as a coherent whole, with each item contributing to both other items and the final objective. If the objective of the meeting can be summarised in about ten lines it will give some idea of the logical order of the items on the agenda. Some general points to be taken into account when constructing an agenda include:

a. Is the early part of the agenda progressive/enthusiastic?
b. The agenda can be 'timed' with the time to be allocated to urgent but unimportant items specified: with practice all items can be 'timed'.
c. Can there be some items early on, on the agenda, which will be well known to most of those taking part? (This encourages participation.)
d. Does it build up to a climax at the end? (An anticlimax should be avoided.)
e. Do 'following' items gain strength and effect from those coming earlier?
f. Are the 'controversial' items timed to coincide with the most conciliatory parts of the meeting?
g. Will meal or tea breaks interfere with or help those items likely to coincide with the breaks?
h. Will the inevitable late-comers or early leavers interfere with the effect of important items?

The agenda should be available before the meeting so that everyone can prepare their contribution and thoughts—thinking on one's feet is often grossly unsatisfactory.

Timing

a. The chairman needs to be in his seat at the time the meeting is due to begin. Poor time-keeping habits tend to grow. Strategies can be adopted to deal with this. Starting meetings on time even if everybody isn't present tends to improve time-keeping at subsequent meetings.
b. Meetings should not drag on merely to legitimate attendance. A short meeting can be favourably received. Long meetings court inattention, discomfort and irritation.
c. Do keep to the stated finishing time. People who leave early assuming a meeting will drag on may be motivated to stay to the end if meetings actually finish at the time given. A stated finishing time allows people to plan other commitments—it also concentrates the mind wonderfully!

Handling personalities

It is a chairman's job to:
a. Inculcate a cooperative attitude
b. Ensure that everybody is treated with respect
c. Deal with one point at a time
d. Avoid argument early on.

Inculcate a co-operative attitude

Merely bringing people together does not mean cooperation. Cooperation means the integration of people, ideas and action in a coordinated way and this calls for listening in a positive way. The manner in which the chairman listens is contagious. Gestures, manners and refraining from other activities are all very important.

Ensure that everybody is treated with respect

Even if one disagrees there are a variety of ways in which this can be expressed e.g.
  (i) 'That's nonsense. I don't believe a word of it. Why don't you read your papers?'
 (ii) 'The point you make might seem valid to you but I disagree, I think.'
(iii) 'Your point is interesting and your position logical, but additional facts might lead to a different conclusion.'
 (iv) 'You have a good point, we'd like to support but.'
    It is important that the chairman aims to:
a. Understand rather than refute
b. Weigh the point rather than the person
c. Achieve progress rather than score points
d. Keep a neutral position.

If one has a lot to say at a meeting then probably someone else should be chairing it—a one man show to an audience is not a meeting.

Deal with one point at a time

At any meeting there are six major roles being played, namely:
a. Opinion giver
b. Opinion seeker

c. Fact giver
d. Fact seeker
e. Tester of feasibility
f. Definer of problem.

Role (a) is the one adopted by most of us most of the time. Roles
(e) and (f) are the ones which characterise the leaders of meetings.
Being aware of this is helpful in keeping to a point and dealing with
it before moving on to the next. The chairman should always
summarise discussion and decisions made before moving on to the
next point.

Avoid argument early on

If someone persists in opposition to a course generally supported
by the others, it is often desirable for the chairman to ask the
meeting if it will agree to a private discussion between the dissenter,
one other interested person and himself, the decision to be reported
to the next meeting. Dissention is thereby removed from the
meeting and often results in a peaceful solution being found. Where
a private discussion is not feasible, the disagreement and dissenter
should be respected and the issue closed, moving on to the next
point before the proceedings are poisoned!

After the meeting

The follow-up is the test of a good meeting.
  Points to be watched for include:

1. Each decision to be implemented should be associated with a
   time and date of completion. A margin on the right of a page
   can be used for this recording.
2. Individuals responsible for implementing decisions should have
   their names clearly recorded in the minutes together with the
   name of the person to whom completion is to be reported.
3. The minutes should be concise—not more than two pages—and
   circulated as quickly as possible. They could be typed and
   copied whilst the meeting is wound up.
4. Progress should be reported at the next meeting, this is
   important if people are to feel accountable.

At this point one reaches full circle. What follows one meeting
precedes the next. In this context the significance of asking questions in the right way becomes important. For written questions the
following points are useful.

a. Put a heading on the paper which catches the eye and interest of the person receiving it. This not only helps in achieving action, but it helps identify the paper and assists filing.
b. Be concise.
c. Seek commitment. For 'no' answers ask for specific reasons.
d. Ask for confirmation of set targets and dates.
e. Attempt to make the question as meaningful to the person being asked for information as the person seeking information.
f. If a question is directed at a number of people they should all see the replies.
g. For circulated questions/information include a circulation list.
h. Put a reminder in your diary when such follow-up is to be initiated.

The chairman will find the execution of these duties slightly eased if he bears the previous sections in mind. For instance, in chairing discussion, it is useful to be able to follow the problem solving structure of organising discussion to:

1. Collecting information and describing the problem, and only then
2. Make sense of it and only often that
3. Let the discussion move onto considering solutions and strategies.

You may wish to photocopy this section and give it to the person who chairs some of your own meetings. This is, of course, illegal and infringes the copyright rules, so lend them the book.

CONFLICT AND NEGOTIATION

Winning and losing

On occasion the occupational therapist is offered the chance to be in conflict with someone else. You can always decline this invitation of it does not suit you. There is no point in entering a conflict or fight if you are going to lose. Of course, you may be prepared to lose in one area if there is a trade off somewhere else, or there will be a definite benefit in the longer term. Indeed, on matters of principle you will fight because not to fight would be truly to lose whereas to lose that particular battle is, in fact, to win.

Let us, then, look at a framework for conflict and at strategies of negotiation. Galvin Whitaker says that one should always be able to anser these two questions before proceeding: 'What is the price of winning?' You may recall Lt Calley, charged with the massacre of Vietnamese villagers, answered in his defence, 'in order to save the village we had to destroy it.' There are many times when the price of winning is too great and under those circumstances it is better not to fight.

The second question is: 'Whose will will prevail?' If the odds are against you, do not fight! Wait until the odds are in your favour. The more important the issue the more important it is to act with circumspection, discretion and success.

There is a famous parable told to illustrate the problems of conflict called 'Prisoner's dilemma'. Jake and Bill meet up one day and decide to rob a bank. They are exceedingly good at robbing banks. They do the job and get back home and into bed by 3 a.m. Suddenly there is a knock on the door, 'Open up in the name of the Law' comes the demand. To cut a longer story short, they are taken down to the Police Station, put in separate cells, and after an hour or so, the Inspector visits each one of them in turn and says, 'We know you did it, lad. Now do us a good turn and do yourself a favour, turn Queen's evidence on the other fellow and we'll drop the charge against you.'

The dilemma is as follows: if they both deny the charge, they both get off because the Police cannot make the charge stick. If one of them grasses on the other whilst that other is still denying the charge, then the grass gets off and the other one takes the full rap— and, further, the grass does not have to share the stashed loot with him. But, if they both grass, then there is evidence on them both and they both go down, although not for as long as if they took the sole rap. Figure 12.2. shows the dilemma.

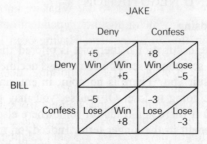

Fig. 12.2 The win–lose game in negotiation.

What would you do? If you can be absolutely sure of Jake, then, as Bill, you deny the charge. Or if you are sure that he will not grass on you, then you can grass on him and get his share of the haul.

But if you deny it and he grasses on you then he gets your share. It is a pretty little game to play over ten rounds because once one person—say Bill—breaks faith, then Jake is likely to grass back on him because that way he will lose less by doing so than he would lose through trusting Bill. Once one person starts playing about and acting greedy it is very difficult to regain the top left hand box again—and that is a chronic problem, even if the people involved are colleagues involved in, for example, occupational therapy.

We have, then, the Win/Win Box, the Win/Lose Boxes and the Lose/Lose Box. As long as both occupational therapist and charge nurse are working together on a Win/Win strategy there is a basic positive pay-off for them both, they make five points each and every day and take home 25 units of well-being and satisfaction at the end of the week. We can, of course, imagine a situation where they distrust each other and expect the worst of each other and play safe in the Lose/Lose box in which the most that they can lose is three points—and they just might make an eight now and again. At the end of the week this war of attrition will have taken its toll in a quiet and persistent fashion but the most they can lose is $3 \times 5 = 15$ and that is certainly better than having risked the Win/Lose box and lost each day thus losing a total of $5 \times 5 = 25$ points down. In the first instance they were chosing a strategy whereby to maximise their gains: in the second it was the strategy of minimising their losses.

The problem, of course, is what to do when you were working with someone in order to maximise your gains and suddenly they land you a minus five. Suddenly you are let down by your colleague and you need to work out what to do. What we know is that there is an inexorable logic which pulls interdependent outcomes such as this one through the Win/Lose box. Having been let down once, why not a second time? Should I punish them and get my own back when next I have a chance? If I say nothing, does that give the impression that I can be pushed around?

Fortunately, occupational therapists do not work in separate cells and so there is the possibility of discussing the matter with your colleague who might have made a mistake, might have also got a minus five from the interaction since a third party had let her down; or she might indeed have been trying to pull a fast one on your and you need to show her that this road leads to both of you faring worse in the long term, even if in the short term there is some advantage for her. Everyone always lets someone else down every day—it is important to devise a structure and understanding that keeps you off the slippery Win/Lose slope that leads to Lose/Lose. You might like to take a moment and think about the dilemma of the situation in which you 'can win the battle at the cost of the war'.

You might like now to consider how you would recognise a situation in which your 'colleague' was so mean and wretched that you have to work a 'Minimise your Losses Strategy'. (Consider also that life is too short to waste in a Lose/Lose game—when I talk with people who have left unsatisfactory work-places they usually say 'I should have left a couple of years earlier'; learn from their experience, if the writing is on the wall, recognise it before you get exhausted!)

Figure 12.3 describes the two basic dimensions of a conflict situation. The mode of resolution of the conflict depends upon (1) the assertiveness of each party in pursuing their own goals and (2) how cooperative each person is in pursuing the goals of the other party. The final mode of resolution depends upon where each person is on each of these two dimensions. Let us first consider Sue; if she is assertive and cooperative, then she is likely to be offering a collaborative solution: if she is neither concerned about her own goals nor Janet's goals, then she will offer to avoid any conflict: if she is concerned about her own goals but not about Janet's then she will offer a competition between the two of them . . . and so on. Janet's position is similarly identified. The outcome of their conflict will be a product of how their stances and invitations to each other mesh together. The style Janet adopts interacts with the style Sue favours and the actual way in which they deal with this situation is a product of the two styles in interaction. You might

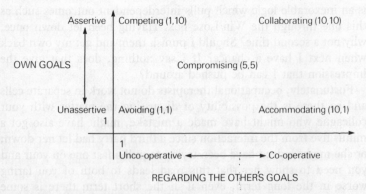

Fig. 12.3 Gains in different styles of negotiation (Blake & Mouton, 1964).

like to consider some of the issues that feature in a couple of your relationships and work out how this model fits what actually happens. Remember that if this is a relationship with a colleague then the outcome affects your patients, not just yourselves—and recognise how concern for the other person's goals makes it more likely that—in the long term as in the prisoner's dilemma—individually and collectively you will benefit!

Strategies

There are a number of different ways in which a conflict of interests can be conducted. It is very important to be able to determine which is the structure of resolution that is most appropriate to the particular situation.

1. Conversion

My response to our conflict of interests—or beliefs—is to attempt to convert you to my way of thinking. I attempt this through force of argument, personality or threat. There are certainly times when this is effective and appropriate but it can also serve to make the conflict worse and generate a lot of bad feeling that could be very unfortunate in the long run.

2. Joint problem solving

This is where we both recognise the situation we are in and set about working together on a joint goal that will permit both of us to gain our own goals en route. We put our cards on the table and try to understand the other's position and, working together, hope to find a resolution in which we both get all that we want. For instance, instead of competing for certain limited resources, we decide to work together to increase the total amount of resources so that we can then split them up each getting as much, or more, than would have been the case had we disputed for them. However, if your protagonist does not want to work with you in this way, you may have put yourself at a grave disadvantage and may well end up merely giving in stages! A second problem is that if it is not possible to (in the above example) get extra resources or to get a consensus between the various parties, the conflict just goes on in an inconclusive way causing much delay and frustration.

3. Negotiation

This is a more expensive structure than problem solving since it involves the trading of concessions. In problem solving you hope to make no concessions but in negotiation the exchange of concessions is the essential component of the conversations towards resolution. Many people feel nervous about negotiation—they fear being out-manoeuvred and taken advantage of by the other person and therefore refuse to negotiate. Where problem solving is inappropriate, conversion is ineffective and negotiation is not available then all that is left is a stand-off with neither person getting even a bit of what they need or want.

There is a structure of four phases in negotiation and if you are aware of the sequence of phases and how to manage each one it is likely that you will be able to negotiate in a way that brings satisfaction to you—and also to the other person. Remember, if the other person feels that they have been taken advantage of they will not work well with you.

The stages are as follows:

1. Prepare

Define your objective and work out your preferred and your minimum positions so that you can identify what concessions you are prepared to exchange. Work out what information you need and get it—especially about what the others want of the deal. Then prepare yourself a simple strategy for the following:

2. Argue and discuss

State your opening (and realistic) position and listen to his. Test out assumptions you have made and exchange information and learn what is important to him as well as what is important to you, *and* signal your interest in continuing to talk. 'There are our standard charges . . .', 'that would be very difficult to agree to . . .' and '. . . as things stand' are all ways of signalling that the situation is open to further negotiation!

3. Propose

You next move to making suggestions in order to advance the negotiation. 'What if . . .', '. . . could consider . . . may be'. Do not interrupt, just listen to the suggestions, question them, summarise them and offer counter-proposals until you both feel you have an idea of the width of the other person's thoughts and limits. Then construct a 'package'—re-present the original proposal in a different form in the light of what you have learnt in the above discussions.

4. Bargain

This only happens after the preparatory phases have been explored. This is where, having got a good idea of what is important to the other person, you can start to trade concessions. The formula is clear; *if* you will do X, *then* I will concede Y; state the condition before the offer and never concede anything without something being given in return. Bit by bit the two parties move closer together (or one party realises that no realistic and satisfactory deal is possible) and eventually one person moves to the 'close' by trading a final concession for a deal: '*If* you will throw in Z *then* we have a deal'.

And finally you both agree what was agreed, summarise and record the resolution so that when you need to re-negotiate it some time in the future you both know where you are starting from.

Do not rush negotiations. Take your time and take pauses to think. Do not get to the bargaining stage too soon or you may well find that you miss opportunities to create a deal that satisfies both yourself and the other person—with whom you probably have to work for the next few years!

To review this immediate passage, there are several different structures for organising the resolution of conflicts and differences of interest. It is important to identify which structure is appropriate for any situation so that the most fruitful resolution can be found. There is no special merit in any one structure but there is a grave danger of finding yourself doing one approach when the other person is using a different one.

The key note in this section has been that it is legitimate and necessary to recognise that the handling of conflict and the selection of strategies for negotiation are professional tasks and need to be thought about and planned like all other interventions in one's professional life. If you count up the percentage of the working week spent in such negotiations, and if you consider how these bits balance those that are more directly related to your clients, then you realise that you get a third of your money for exercising these particular skills!

But, before we move to the final section, a very useful quotation taken from *Illuminatus* by A Wilson & R. Shea (for redundant read 'rigid'):

> People exist on a spectrum from the most redundant to the most flexible. The latter, unless they are thoroughly trained in psychodynamics, are always at a disadvantage to the former in social interactions. The redundant do not change their script; the flexible continually keep changing, trying to find a way of relating constructively. Eventually the flexible ones find the 'power' gambit, and communication, of a sort, is possible. They are now on the set created by the redundant person, and they act out his or her script.
>
> The steady exponential growth of bureaucracy is not due to Parkinson's Law alone. The State, by making itself even more redundant, incorporates more people into its set and forces them to follow its script.

Power, responsibility and information

There is a constant conservative tendency of people and organisations to attribute the cause of someone's behaviour to their personality. Some years back I ran some research on this subject and had my suspicions confirmed: when asked why someone does a thing—such as shout at a dog—people replied that the man shouted at the dog because he was that sort of man. When asked why they might shout at a dog they attributed the cause to external factors—such as the dog's behaviour. The world is a simpler, more manageable place if we just see the cause for a person's behaviour in their 'personality', even though we know perpectly well that if we were to do it—or someone we know well were to do it—we would look beyond their personality for an explanation of their behaviour.

When there is a difficulty or failing in part of an organisation, the organisation will tend to attribute the cause to the personalities of the people involved or responsible. However, if you speak with the persons involved, it is often the case that they can identify other reasons—such as a poor line of communication, lack of secretarial assistance, a qualitative change in the severity of the handicap of the client group etc.—which have caused the pressure and the failure. The organisation will attribute the cause to the 'personalities' of those involved since it can follow that diagnosis with the prescription that *they* should change. Were the organisation to realise that it was a structurally induced failure, then the *organisation* would have to change—which is less readily perceived by those in a position to effect it. You can probably identify certain posts in your organisation in which, whoever occupies it, the work is impaired and the occupant blamed. Such posts have a high turn-over but each occupant gets blamed in their turn for a structurally induced handicap. Avoid such a post.

You will remember from the discussion of groups that the individual who is expressing his boredom and dissatisfaction can either be seen as a disruptive personality or as the member expressing the group's malfunction. It is the same thing.

Dorothy and Galvin Whitaker, respectively Professor of Social Work at York University and Reader in Management Studies at Leeds University, recommend the following diagnostic structure for examining the performance of a task in an organisation. It is derived from a psychoterapeutic model of effectiveness.

$$\text{Task} \rightarrow (\text{Power} \equiv \text{Responsibility} \equiv \text{Information}) \times \text{Competence}$$

Thus, in considering the work performed by a staff member, first it is necessary to identify the specific tasks that they perform and to check whether this information has been made available to the worker. It is common to find people employed on one job-description and yet expected to fulfil a different one.

The effectiveness of the work performance to this task is dependent upon four further factors. The natural conservatism of organisations leads one to first enquire after the competence of the staff member and, as suggested earlier, to ask no further. However, this present model obliges one to recognise the following dynamic as being the modifier of such competence in practice.

The amount of responsibility allocated to a worker must be balanced by a commensurate amount of power and also a commen-surate amount of information (information about both his own role and duties and also the wider context of the purpose of the work). Responsibility and power without sufficient information will make the best of workers a menace to his colleagues: the best truck driver in a powerful vehicle for which he is responsible is dangerous if his windscreen is whitewashed. Another example often quoted is of certain senior administrators who have undoubted qualities, responsibility and power, but who do not actually know what is happening in certain portions—operational portions—of their organisation. Should they be sacked for incompetence or do we look to see how to supply the necessary information? We will then know to sack them if they still cannot manage their jobs.

Responsibility and information without commensurate level of power renders the worker helpless. Either the accountability/

responsibility must be reduced or the discretion and power must be increased because until that time it is unlikely that this helpless worker will be able to perform the tasks adequately.

Power and information without responsibility is another imbalanced and destructive situation, although not as crippling as the previous examples. This can occur when a receptionist achieves influence on the informal communication network and, as usual, knows more of what is happening around an organisation than anyone else: if she gets bored or annoyed she is in a position to guide affairs without being responsible for the outcome.

We look at the occupational therapist's performance and we ask about the external situational factors such as how clearly the task is defined, how the power, information and responsibility factors are balanced before we presume to assess her competence. The approach also allows us to diagnose an organisation by taking different sections and different posts within them and asking these questions rather than glibly saying that of course the occupational therapy department is a mess, look at the head occupational therapist, or 'no wonder that psychiatrist is a disaster to his patients, look at the bumbling arrogant way the visits are arranged'. Instead, you ask the questions and refrain from making personal attributions until it is appropriate, if it is appropriate.

You will find this equation invaluable; commit it to your memory, use it often and look for the situational factors before you start criticizing others. Maybe others might do this for you, too. Maybe.

REFERENCES

Blake R R, Mouton J S 1964 The managerial grid. Gulf Publishing Company, Texas

Schutz W C 1958 FIRO: A 3D theory of interpersonal behaviour. Rinehart, New York

Shea R, Wilson A 1977 The golden apple. Sphere, New York

Index

Reich, 183
Reinforcement, 133, 135, 145
Referral, 186
Regression, 58
Relationship
  with patients, 89, 191
  with families, 232
Relaxation, 41, 150, 166, 170, 202
Repression, 31, 183
Responsibility, 264
Richard D, 61
Roberts K, 224
Roberston J N, 180
Rogers C, 13, 73, 74, 76, 82, 132
Rokeach M, 91
Roles, 15, 29, 54, 58
Role play, 124, 150, 166, 192,
  238
Role reversal, 195
Rowan, 73
Rutter M, 37, 133

Scharfetter C, 7, 17
Schizophrenia, 5, 148, 209
Schools, 206
Sculpting, 195
Self, 83, 85
  actualisation, 78, 81, 132
  care, 212
  concept, 55
  determination, 107
  esteem, 206
  monitoring, 122
  report, 121
  styling, 227
  theories of, 74
Seligman J, 33
Sex role, 110
Sexual dysfunction, 42, 159
Shutz W, 241
Siller J, 67
Simulation, 125
Skinner F, 11
Social activities, 215, 219
  anxiety, 116
  assessment, 121–126
  competence, 144
  difficulty, 119–120
  drama, 193
  inadequacy, 145
  incongruity, 61
  learning, 110, 111, 112, 133
  problems, 231
  roles, 115
  rules, 115

situations, 114–117
  skills, 213, 142
  skills training, 131–155
  support, 16
Sociodrama, 193
Socialisation, 93, 110
Sociology, 91
Spitz R N, 35
Sport, 216
Stang and Wrightsman, 107
Stature, 66
Status, 237
Stigma, 66, 231
Stress, 26, 29
Stuart Mill J, 97
Sublimation 31, 183
Suicide, 42
Superego, 10
Symbols (in drama), 195
Sympathetic nervous system, 30
Systematic desensitisation, 41

Targets (see goals)
Tasks, 15, 115, 244
Taulbee and Wright, 44, 49
Tension, 26
Thatcher D, 34
Therapeutic skills, 183
Thorndyke E, 11
Thought, 16, 19, 22
Totman R, 56, 60, 61
Tranquillisers, 41 (see Drugs)
Trait theory, 111
Transactional analysis, 149
Transference, 182
Trauma, 35, 55
Trombley and Scott, 235
Trower P, 140, 166
Trust, 196

Unconscious mechanisms, 30
Utilitarianism, 97

Values, 90, 95–98
Van Hassett V, 150
Verbal ability, 19 (see also
  Communication)
Video, 125, 154
Voluntary work, 210, 223
Vulnerable personalities, 43

Wakefulness, 20
Walton H J, 35
Watson, 33
Webber M, 221